I see in Dr. Max G⸱⸱⸱⸱ ⸱⸱⸱⸱ ⸱⸱⸱ ⸱⸱⸱⸱ ⸱⸱⸱⸱⸱⸱⸱⸱ nt geniuses in the his⸱⸱⸱⸱⸱ ⸱⸱ ⸱⸱⸱⸱⸱⸱⸱⸱. Many of his basic ideas have been adopted without having his name connected with them. He has achieved more than seemed possible under adverse conditions. He leaves a legacy which commands attention and that will assure him his due place. Those whom he cured will attest to the truth of his ideas.

—Albert Schweitzer

For over thirty years I have recommended the Gerson metabolic therapy to persons fighting serious illness, and have never once had cause to regret it. This new Gerson manual is comprehensive, up to date, exhaustively referenced, and very well written. It fully explains the therapy as it instructs on exactly how to do it. Most importantly, *Healing Diabetes: The Gerson Way* is about healing diabetes, which is supposedly incurable. Don't let anyone use that word with you: there is much more available than surgery, drugs and still more drugs. This excellent book is a compendium of knowledge, based on decades of proven effectiveness, that you will want to share with everyone you know.

—Andrew W. Saul
Author of *Doctor Yourself and Fire Your Doctor*

Healing Diabetes

THE GERSON WAY

Healing Diabetes

THE GERSON WAY

BASED ON THE RESEARCH OF

Dr. Max Gerson

Charlotte Gerson

Gerson Health Media

Gerson Health Media
316 Mid Valley Center #230
Carmel, CA 93923
www.gersonmedia.com

For more information on books and DVDs about Gerson Therapy or other health topics, go to www.GersonMedia.com.

ISBN-13: 978-1-937920-10-4
ISBN-10: 1-937920-10-0

Printed and bound in the United States by Sheridan Books, Ann Arbor, MI. This book was printed on recycled paper with 30% PCW.

To contact the Gerson Institute/Cancer Curing Society, please go to www.gerson.org, or call (619) 685-5353.

In Italy, contact Margaret Straus at associazione.gerson@gmail.com.

For other European countries, contact the Gerson Health Centre in Hungary at info@gerson.hu.

For an up-to-date list of Gerson Therapy Resources, go to www.gerson.org.

Cover design provided by 1106 Design, Phoenix, AZ (http://1106design.com).

Interior design, editing and production by Joanne Shwed, Backspace Ink, Pacifica, CA (www.backspaceink.com).

Contents

Acknowledgements

This book is above all a tribute to my father, Dr. Max Gerson. He was not just a doctor but a true healer. He deeply understood the basic organization of the incredibly complex and wonderful organism that is the human body, and through his genius he learned how to restore and heal those who were failing. He was not only a healer, but he hoped to bring healing to all the world, to end disease and suffering.

Building on his vast knowledge and experience, we have often been able to bring complete healing, a return of life and health, to those who were once pronounced "incurable" and who faced long years of suffering or death. In this volume, we aim to bring the details of his approach to those who will use it to return to happy and productive lives.

Max and Charlotte Gerson

In the past 50 years, the world has changed, conditions have worsened and the healing knowledge has had to be adapted to these changes. It has taken many people of knowledge, experience and vision to achieve these adaptations. It took many more people to help us to record the infinite details of the Gerson treatment.

It is virtually impossible to thank by name all who were involved in the production of this book. They are the Gerson-trained physicians, the nurses and the helpers who produce the hourly juices—and of vital importance, the dedicated caregivers who carry out the daily routine needed for healing. **The patients, too, are our heroes, disciplined and steady in their adherence to the therapy.** It took those friends, acquaintances and family members who encouraged patients to stay on course and not to give up just because their original doctor gave them a death sentence.

Howard Straus

Margaret Straus

It took my son, Howard Straus, to contribute to this book with uncounted hours of research for references, ideas and suggestions, to put the information on the World Wide Web and to lecture in the United States, Canada and Asia.

It took my daughter, Margaret Straus, whose lectures, seminars, editing, articles and publicity introduced the Gerson Therapy into England, Ireland and Italy, and whose help and encouragement of patients inspired one of our most famous successes, my dear friend, Beata Bishop.

Beata Bishop   **Yvonne Nienstadt**

First as a dedicated patient, rewarded with a dramatic recovery, Beata Bishop helped with her great experience and constructive ideas in editing and improving the structure of this book. Her own book, *A Time to Heal*,[1] in which she described her life-threatening illness and full recovery on the Gerson Therapy, has been translated into eight languages and has presumably saved many lives worldwide.

Twenty years ago, Beata introduced the Gerson Therapy into Hungary, where today there is a growing number of recovered patients. She founded the Hungarian Gerson Support Group, which now has its own residential facility, run by a trained Gerson therapist and supported by sympathetic doctors. In 1993, Beata was one of the founders of the British Gerson Support Group, of which she remains an active member. We are also very grateful to this group for allowing us to use most of the recipes from their publication, *Gerson Gourmet*. Other contributors to the recipe chapter include Yvonne Nienstadt, Susan DeSimone and several recovered Gerson patients.

Charlotte Gerson

It took many, many more people, too numerous to name individually, to help, encourage and support us, psychologically and often financially, to bring this project to fruition. To all of those dedicated supporters continuing Dr. Gerson's healing work—I devote this book with the deepest gratitude.

—Charlotte Gerson
Bonita, California
July 2012

ACKNOWLEDGEMENTS REFERENCE

1.   Beata Bishop, *A Time to Heal,* 2nd edition (Penguin UK, June 1999).

List of Acronyms

CDC	Centers for Disease Control and Prevention
DDT	dichloro-diphenyl-trichloroethane
FDA	[U.S.] Food and Drug Administration
GM	genetically modified
GMO	genetically modified organism
HDL	high-density lipoprotein
HVO	hydrogenated vegetable oil
LDL	low-density lipoprotein
MSG	monosodium glutamate
NCI	[U.S.] National Cancer Institute
WHO	World Health Organization

Introduction

E very year, the problem of obesity increases to the point where it has become worldwide, particularly in the so-called "developed" countries where a large portion of the population consumes fast foods and restaurant meals. **The problem of obesity leading to age-onset (also called type 2 or adult-onset) diabetes and high blood pressure has a new name: "the Metabolic Syndrome."**

It is surprising that India, with its considerable vegetarian population, has an especially high incidence of age-onset diabetes.[1] This phenomenon can most likely be ascribed to the regular consumption of large amounts of extremely sweet snacks and deep-fried, highly seasoned and salted foods.[2]

Furthermore, with increased prosperity and technological advances, people tend to do less physical work. They live in large cities and their higher standard of living has meant increased meat and alcohol consumption. Resorting to junk foods is another relatively recent phenomenon, since these were introduced only some 20-25 years ago.

In Europe, smoking has increased, especially among women. A number of widely prescribed drugs, such as antidepressants and antipsychotics, also contribute to obesity. MSG (monosodium glutamate) is used to make lab animals fat[3] and is now added to some 6,000 food items available in groceries.[4] Restaurant operators, too, have found that people will consume more when MSG is used generously in their recipes.

In many obese people, weight gain leads to age-onset diabetes (the only type of diabetes with which we are concerned in this book). Contrary to what is advertised by pharmaceutical companies and assumed by the public, diabetes is not controlled by drugs.

Norton Hadler, MD, of the University of North Carolina, has stated, "No oral diabetes drug has ever been shown to do anything really good for any patient. No leg, eye, kidney, heart or brain has been spared."[5] This statement illustrates the extensive and devastating organ damage caused by diabetes: blindness, gangrene of the extremities (often requiring amputation), kidney failure leading to dialysis, high blood pressure, nonhealing skin lesions, and nerve damage. **Diabetes is the sixth largest disease killer in the United States.**[6]

It is also false to claim, as the pharmaceutical companies do, that diabetics are insulin resistant. Nathan Pritikin showed in the 1950s that, **in some 85% of diabetics, adequate insulin is available in the bloodstream but is unable to reach the cell.** All cells have specialized insulin receptors that are activated by the penetrating insulin to produce energy. These receptors, Pritikin found, are blocked and coated with cholesterol, so that insulin is unable to reach them.[7]

In other words, age-onset diabetes is a cholesterol problem. That also explains why the Gerson Therapy is so effective. It helps the body remove cholesterol *without* toxic anticholesterol medication, restoring well-being through truly healthy nutrition.

The Gerson Therapy will help the determined person get a quick start on reversing their disease and achieve rapid results.

- In Part I, "An Overview of Diabetes and the Gerson Therapy" (p. 1), Chapters 1 through 5 explain the connection between obesity and diabetes, the causes of each and, by extension, the necessity for correct nutrition and its positive effects.

- In Part II, "The Path to Healing" (p. 63), Chapters 6 through 21 serve as a complete how to guide for the Gerson Therapy and provide the details for the preparation of foods, juices and enema preparation as well as the use of appropriate supplements.

INTRODUCTION REFERENCES

1. Sarah Wild, MB BChir, PhD; Gojka Roglic, MD; Anders Green, MD, PhD, Dr Med Sci; Richard Sicree, MBBS, MPH; Hilary King, MD, DSC. "Global Prevalence of Diabetes: Estimates for the year 2000 and projections for 2030," *Diabetes Care*, 27:5, May 2004. "The crude prevalence rate of diabetes in urban areas is about 9% and that the prevalence in rural areas has also increased to around 3% of the total population. If one takes into consideration that the total population of India is more than 1000 million then one can understand the sheer numbers involved. Taking a urban-rural population distribution of 70:30 and an overall crude prevalence rate of around 4%, at a conservative estimate, India is home to around 40 million diabetics and this number is thought to give India the dubious distinction of being home to the largest number of diabetics in any one country." The Indian Task Force On Diabetes Care In India (www.diabetesindia.com/diabetes/itfdci.htm).

2. J. Carey, "Surprising New Diabetes Data," *BusinessWeek Magazine*, Feb. 6, 2008. In a recent *New England Journal of Medicine* commentary, Dr. Clifford Rosen, chair of the Food & Drug Administration advisory committee that evaluated one such drug (GlaxoSmithKline's Avandia), wrote that "the two largest randomized, placebo-controlled trials in patients with type 2 diabetes, the United Kingdom Prospective Diabetes Study and the University Group Diabetes Program, failed to find a significant reduction on cardiovascular events even with excellent glucose control."

3. John E. and T. M. Erb, *The Slow Poisoning of America* (available on-line at https://www.spofamerica.com).

4. FoodFacts.com: "It is now estimated that over 6,000 food and drink products worldwide contain this popular artificial sweetener." (http://blog.foodfacts.com/index.php/2009/09/08/aspartame-nutrition-facts). The Aspartame Information Center quotes 6,000 products as containing aspartame (www.aspartame.org/aspartame_products.html).

5. Note 2 (Carey), supra.

6. "Leading Causes of Death," U.S. Centers for Disease Control and Prevention final 2009 statistics (http://www.cdc.gov/nchs/fastats/lcod.htm).

7. Ross Horne, *The Health Revolution* (Avalon Beach, NSW, Australia: Happy Landings, Pty. Ltd., 1980), pp. 313-314. Early stages of diabetes (type 2) are characterized by adequate, and often excessive, production of insulin, leading to tissue damage from hyperinsulinemia. Thus, the

majority of type 2 diabetics were, at least initially, oversupplied with endogenic insulin, which could not be utilized by the cells.

PART I

An Overview of Diabetes and the Gerson Therapy

CHAPTER 1

What is Diabetes?

3

Type 1 Diabetes

Type 1 diabetes—also called juvenile diabetes—results from the failure of the pancreas' Islets of Langerhans to produce adequate insulin. This may damage blood vessels, nerves, kidneys, the retina and, during pregnancy, it may damage the developing fetus.

Obese people are more prone to this type of diabetes as are people with sedentary lifestyles. **Juvenile diabetes in children is usually the result of an infection that appears to be a long, drawn-out flu but is actually a pancreatitis.** It is incorrectly diagnosed as "autoimmune" destruction of the Islets of Langerhans. The actual destruction occurs from the infectious response to viruses, and breakdown products of the Islets are found in the blood; however, they are not caused by "autoimmune" action but by damage due to viral infection.

Orthodox treatments for this type of diabetes with drugs can result in kidney damage, renal failure needing dialysis, coronary vascular disease and reduced resistance to infections. Frequent problems are ulcerations of the toes, feet, and legs, which may require amputation. In most cases of diabetes type 1, insulin injections are required permanently.

Symptoms include excessive urination (thirst), kidney damage and skin breakdown. Lifelong medication will probably be required.

Type 2 Diabetes

Type 2 diabetes—also known as "diabetes mellitus," "mature-onset," "adult-onset," "age-onset" or "noninsulin-dependent" diabetes—comprises roughly 95% of the diabetes in the United States. *Taber's Cyclopedic Dictionary, 17th Edition* (1993) presumes it to be a "chronic disorder of the carbohydrate metabolism" that is "incurable" but treatable to prolong life and ameliorate symptoms.[1] Whereas type 1 diabetes is characterized by inadequate production of insulin, type 2 diabetics often produce adequate, even excessive insulin, but the insulin is not properly used by the cells.

The symptoms of diabetes mellitus are characterized by alternating episodes of hypoglycemia and hyperglycemia.[2] **It may also be caused by insulin that is not well absorbed** and by damage produced by drugs, such as corticosteroids, statins, certain diuretics or birth control pills.

Type 2 diabetes includes symptoms such as excess body weight, which are rapidly becoming a worldwide problem, specifically in the so-called "developed countries." **In these areas, a large proportion of the population is eating fast foods, restaurant meals and sweet snacks and drinking more alcohol,** leading to obesity, diabetes, high blood pressure and other serious breakdowns of bodily functions.

An unhealthy accumulation of body fat (obesity) "is the most common metabolic/nutritional disease in the US. More than 50% of the adult population is overweight. It is more common in women, minorities and in the poor."[2] The problem becomes more severe because "overweight individuals have an increased risk of developing diabetes, hypertension (high blood pressure), heart disease, stroke and cancer."[3]

It is surprising that India, with a largely vegetarian population due to its religion, has an especially high incidence of type 2 diabetes. On closer examination, however, the high rate of diabetes seems to be due to the consumption of large amounts of extremely sweet snacks along with deep-fried, highly seasoned and salted foods, generously provided with fats and oil. Furthermore, as people become more prosperous due to technology, they tend to do less physical work. They live in cities and are exposed to junk foods that became available some 20-25 years ago. They eat more meat (chicken, pork and lamb) and drink sweet bottled juices. They also consume more alcohol. In Europe smoking has also seriously increased. These new habits and lifestyles influence the body's ability to adjust and they speed up its breakdown.

Thus, the total change of lifestyle that has occurred during the last century points us clearly to the reason for weight gain, diabetes and high blood pressure. **Once we understand the reason (the cause) of a problem, the solution presents itself.** In order to overcome the problem and cure the ensuing disease, **we have to return to the lifestyle of an earlier age by consuming simple, organic food without toxic residue, addi-**

tives or salt, no animal products and raw or freshly prepared as much as possible.

This method (the Gerson Therapy) has produced surprisingly rapid cures of diabetes (type 2) and the entire Metabolic Syndrome. It has also led to the loss of excess weight without cravings or hunger.

Dangerous Diabetes Drugs That Do Not Work

"A large-scale study at Duke University School of Medicine, published in the *New England Journal of Medicine* (April 22, 2010)[4] showed that despite serious risks and dangerous side effects, diabetes drugs offer few benefits and simply don't live up to their claims." The report also states that "practically all anti-diabetic drugs result in weight gain and eventual total dependency upon insulin injections (Krentz, Nichols, and Gomez-Caminero) in two recent articles published in *Current Medical Research Opinion and Diabetes Obesity Metabolism.*"[5]

Robert Califf of the Duke study said, "This is a sobering confirmation of the need to continue to focus on lifestyle improvements."[6]

A case in point was quoted: "Consider the drug Avandia, once the most popular diabetes drug in the world, which was found in **2007** to dramatically increase the risk of heart attacks and death. It took the FDA until November **2011** to finally pull Avandia from the U.S. market.

"Actos, another popular diabetes drug, has its own array of ugly side effects, including average weight gain of nearly nine pounds and a high risk of dangerous and possibly deadly fluid buildups … Some researchers have linked this drug to bladder cancer."[7] [Emphasis added.]

Harmless Spice That Can Help Diabetes

Turmeric, an Asian spice found in many curries, was tested and showed that it does prevent or control type 2 diabetes. Dr. Tortoriello, with resident Stuart Weisberg, MD, PhD, and Rudolph Leibel, MD, endocrinologist and co-director of the Naomi Berrie Diabetes Center, found among other advantages that "obese mice fed turmeric showed significantly reduced inflammation in fat tissue and liver compared to controls."[8] Their findings are in the soon-be-published paper, "Endocrinology," and were presented at ENDO 2008, the Endocrine Society's annual meeting in San Francisco.

Turmeric has no known side effects, even in high doses. Turmeric— and its active antioxidant ingredient curcumin—reverses many of the inflammatory and metabolic problems associated with obesity, according to Dr. Tortoriello and his colleagues.

CHAPTER 1 REFERENCES

1. *Taber's Cyclopedic Medical Dictionary, 17th Edition* (Philadelphia: F. A. Davis Company, 1993), pp. 532-3.
2. *Taber's Cyclopedic Medical Dictionary* (Philadelphia: F. A. Davis Company, 2001), p. 579.
3. Ibid., p. 1504.
4. Ibid.
5. *New England Journal of Medicine* (NEJMoa1001121)
6. *Journal of American Medical Association* (JAMA2010:303(14) 2010:405)
7. Note 5, supra.
8. **Avandia:** (http://articles.cnn.com/2010-02-20/health/avandia.study_1_ avandia-diabetes-drug-glaxosmithkline?_s=PM:HEALTH) "Senate report links diabetes drug Avandia to heart attacks, February 20, 2010" (http:// www.finance.senate.gov/newsroom/chairman/release/?id=bc56b552-efc5-4706-968d-f7032d5cd2e4). February 20, 2010, Grassley, Baucus Release Committee Report on Avandia.
   Actos: (http://www.fda.gov/Safety/MedWatch/SafetyInformation/ SafetyAlertsforHumanMedicalProducts/ucm226257.htm). Actos (pioglitazone): "Ongoing Safety Review—Potential Increased Risk of Bladder Cancer" [UPDATED 08/04/2011] "The U.S. Food and Drug Administration (FDA) is informing the public that the Agency has approved updated drug labels for the pioglitazone-containing medicines to include safety information that the use of pioglitazone for more than one year may be associated with an increased risk of bladder cancer." [UPDATED 06/15/2011] "Use of the diabetes medication Actos (pioglitazone) for more than one year may be associated with an increased risk of bladder cancer. Information about this risk will be added to the Warnings and Precautions section of the label for pioglitazone-containing

medicines. The patient Medication Guide for these medicines will also be revised to include information on the risk of bladder cancer."

9. http://www.ens-newswire.com/ens/jun2008/2008-06-20-091.html

CHAPTER 2

A Quick Overview of the Gerson Therapy for Diabetes

W hile eating should always be a pleasurable experience, the present-day stress on "fun foods" is a dangerous practice. The basic reason for eating, namely the support of the extremely complex human body and mind, seems to have been lost. Worse, the "fun foods" are often seriously processed, devoid of vitamins and minerals and loaded with fats and salt, such as in deep-fried foods, thus promoting obesity with the resulting diabetes!

It is not surprising that obesity contributes seriously to the incidence of diabetes since it also involves excessive consumption of cholesterol: meat products, deep-fried foods, butter and shortening, eggs, cheese, etc. According to the latest release by the Centers for Disease Control and Prevention (CDC), "more than one-third of U.S. adults (35.7%) are obese."[1]

Still more serious, according to a recent release by the American Institute for Cancer Research, obesity causes more than 100,000 cases of cancer every year.[2]

Since the Gerson Therapy eliminates all cholesterol, it deals extremely well with the Metabolic Syndrome. **In a large percentage of the age-**

onset diabetics that are seen in the Gerson clinic, age-onset diabetes clears in an astounding 90% of those patients within 10 days to two weeks, along with a sharp drop in cholesterol and high blood pressure (without drugs). With its sodium restriction, the therapy also causes patients to lose edema, thus producing a considerable weight loss as well for the obese patient.

The therapy provides a start for a permanent cure if the patient carries on the treatment for some months to fully restore the body. Here is the cure for diabetes, obesity and high blood pressure.

To get started:

- **Cut out all salt and/or salted foods.** Salt (sodium) attracts fluid into the tissues because it tends to be toxic and the body defends itself by binding water to the cells to reduce the toxic effect. As salt is eliminated and potassium starts to prevail, the water is excreted and weight is lost! Eating fresh, organic, vegetarian items brings potassium into the tissues. This causes sodium along with retained fluid to be excreted.

- **Eat vegetarian, high-fiber vegetables and fruit.** These will appease appetite and help to move bowels. Animal products contain no fiber. Keep a platter of fresh, raw foods within easy reach. Include celery sticks, green or red sweet pepper strips, tomato slices (or cherry tomatoes), green onions and possibly a few raw apple slices.

- **Eat the special Gerson soup to round out meals.** It is highly satisfying and its valuable ingredients help flush sodium and other toxic substances from the kidneys. (See "Special Soup or Hippocrates Soup," p. 108, in Chapter 11, "Preparing Food and Juices—The Basic Rules.")

- **Eat a good-sized potato once a day.** Use the Gerson recipe for a nice tomato sauce (with no butter or gravy). Eat no deep-fried potatoes or any other fried items as they are loaded with fats and oils as well as salt. Bake potatoes or boil them in their jackets. Use a vinegar (or lemon) dressing with a little flaxseed oil and make a tasty potato salad (or other vegetable salad) with onions, garlic, radishes and/or other treats. (See Chapter 22, "Recipes," p. 165.)

- **Cut out ALL fast foods.** These contain salt, often MSG, fats and frequently sugars. Eat fresh, organic, raw salads and freshly prepared, unsalted vegetables.

- **Cut out all MSG and MSG-containing foods.** This toxic drug is added to a large number of processed foods, often under different names. Eat fresh, organic foods in place of processed items. Restaurants, too, add MSG to their meals to tempt their customers to eat more, so don't eat out!

- **Drink four or more glasses of green juice and/or apple/carrot juice for vitamins, minerals and enzymes.** These juices satisfy hunger and overcome cravings so that the apparently restricted diet is more than adequate in nutrients! Carrots also contain good protein, as do potatoes, oatmeal and many vegetables.

The daily menu looks like this:

Breakfast

- Oatmeal (prepared without milk or salt) with raw or stewed fruit sauce

- One 8-ounce glass of freshly pressed organic grapefruit juice

- Snacks from a fresh vegetable platter

- One or two glasses of juice

Lunch

- Hippocrates Soup (see "Special Soup or Hippocrates Soup," p. 108, in Chapter 11, "Preparing Food and Juices—The Basic Rules").

- Large, raw salad with as many salads, greens, radishes, green onions and tomatoes as possible. Add raw grated garlic to dressing.

- Red beet salad

- One or two vegetable(s), freshly cooked, unsalted

- Fresh fruit, raw or stewed, with apples, melon, pears and plums

- One 8-ounce glass of juice (apple/carrot or green)

- **Snacks and juice**

Dinner

- Hippocrates Soup

- Large salad (similar to lunch)

- Potato, as salad, baked or boiled in jacket

- Vegetable salad (beet, string bean, celery knob)

- Freshly cooked vegetable(s)

- Fresh fruit (similar to lunch)

- Juice (apple/carrot or green)

- **Take a nice, long (about 30 minutes) walk**

- **Avoid drinking water.** At bedtime, provide a thermos with herb tea so that liquid is available if the person is thirsty at night or early in the morning. Adding lemon to taste is suggested. Sweetening with Stevia is permitted; avoid all other sugar substitutes, especially NutraSweet®, Equal®, Spoonful® and Splenda®.

- Perform **at least one coffee enema per day!**

As you will find out later in the book, coffee enemas are an important part of the Gerson Therapy and should not be avoided. Admittedly by western standards, enemas are an odd treatment and we find that patients will try to pass on doing them; however, you must understand they are a vital part of your healing process. Elements in the coffee, when introduced rectally, force the liver to produce large amounts of bile that is then flushed into colon, taking with it deadly chemicals and toxins.

Following the above program usually produces results within a week, two at most. The person not only notes satisfying, even surprising, weight loss, but this therapy almost immediately reduces high blood pressure (if it was elevated), so that drugs can be discontinued. Blood sugar, too, goes down promptly and patients feel better. The elimination of animal foods reduces cholesterol, so that patients can also decrease, and shortly eliminate, anticholesterol drugs.

CHAPTER 2 REFERENCES

1. Centers for Disease Control and Prevention, "Adult Obesity Facts" (2010) (http://www.cdc.gov/obesity/data/adult.html).
2. (http://www.aicr.org/press/press-releases/media-advisory-cancer-group-finds-excess-body-fat-alone-causes-more-than-100000-cancers-in-us.html) "For Immediate Release: November 4, 2009, Contact: Glen Weldon 202-328-7744 x221, Media Advisory: Cancer Group Finds Excess Body Fat Alone Causes More Than 100,000 Cancers in U.S., Presents Latest Scientific Evidence on Adverse Impact of Obesity On Cancer Diagnosis and Survival. WASHINGTON, DC — On the heels of new estimates that obesity-related diseases contribute $147 billion to the nation's health care bill, the American Institute for Cancer Research (AICR) is taking aim at the large number of life-threatening cancers that are preventable through effective weight management. In conjunction with its Annual Research Conference on Food, Nutrition, Physical Activity and Cancer in Washington, **AICR will hold a news conference on November 5 to present new, evidence-based estimates that excess body fat alone is responsible for more than 100,000 cancer cases annually in the U.S.,** including cancers of the endometrium, esophagus, pancreas, kidney, gallbladder, breast and colon/rectum. At the same time, AICR will address the implications of alarmingly low rates of awareness of the obesity/cancer

link among the public and present the latest data linking obesity with poorer outcomes both during and after cancer treatment." [Emphasis added.]

CHAPTER 3

The Connection Between Diabetes and Being Overweight

Overweight is defined as an "unhealthy accumulation of body fat."[1] A person is considered severely overweight when the body mass exceeds 25 kg/m.[2] It is also described as the most common metabolic disease in the United States. More than 50% of the adult population is overweight.[3]

Some medications (e.g., tricyclic antidepressants, insulin and sulfonylurea agents) may cause patients to gain weight. Medications to enhance weight loss, such as amphetamines or amphetamine-like agents, have had unacceptable side effects (e.g., cardiac valvular injuries with fenfluramine/phentermine, addiction with other anorexiants).[4]

The problem can worsen into "morbid obesity," in which the condition interferes with normal activities, including respiration. **Overweight is considered "morbid" when weight exceeds by 100 pounds the normal average for the individual's age, sex and build.**[5]

Not long ago, excessively overweight people drew curious or critical glances in the street; these days, there are too many of them to receive attention. The rapid worldwide spread of fast-food outlets and the exponentially growing sales of convenience foods have sparked a global epidemic of dangerous excessive bodyweight in all age groups.

The word "morbid" means "of the nature of or indicative of disease." Indeed, the medical dictionary quotes excessive bodyweight as a contributing factor; however, it is more than a contributing factor, often a causative factor, to the following diseases: diabetes (type 2), hypertension and some types of cancer.[6] At the time the dictionary was published (1993), it was estimated that 34 million adults in the United States were overweight.[7]

A more recent statement (2001) by the U.S. CDC[8] declared that almost two-thirds of American adults are overweight. The 1980 figures for excessive weight doubled by 2001[9]; diabetes has increased ninefold since 1958[10] and heart disease remains the #1 disease cause of death.[11]

Worst of all, being overweight has become widespread among children. Fat kids are referred to as "small fries: the offspring of couch potatoes." **Between 1980 and 1994, excessive weight in American children increased by 100%**[12]**; currently, one in four children is excessively overweight, as reported by Frank Booth and Donna Krupa.**[13] Lack of exercise is an important contributory factor to this tragic state of affairs, since—according to the above authors—the average child spends 900 hours a year in school and 1,023 hours watching television.

Children being excessively overweight is particularly dangerous since the child's developing organism is less able to deal with the many complications of gross overweight than that of an adult. **Several British researchers have stated that, for the first time in human history, it will be normal for parents to outlive their offspring.**[14]

A hugely successful recent movie, produced by Morgan Spurlock and called *Super Size Me*, unveiled the truth about the destructive effects of fast food. Spurlock, a healthy 33-year-old man, ate all of his meals at McDonald's for 30 days to find out what this exclusive diet would do to him. Throughout the experiment, he was regularly monitored by gastroenterologist Dr. Daryl Isaacs, who declared that Spurlock was "an extremely healthy person who got very sick eating this McDonald's diet."[15] **At one stage, the doctor even told Morgan Spurlock that his liver had turned into paté and asked him to stop his experiment,** but the moviemaker persisted. At the end of the month, Spurlock reported, "I got desperately ill. My face was splotchy and I had this huge gut. [He gained 25 pounds in 30 days.] My knees started to hurt from the extra weight coming on so quickly. It was amazing and frightening."[16] On top of it all, his liver became toxic, his cholesterol shot up from a low 165 to 230, his libido flagged and he suffered from headaches and depression. Within a few days of beginning his "drive-through diet," Spurlock was vomiting out the window of his car, and doctors who examined him were shocked by how rapidly his entire body deteriorated.

Mothers cannot be solely blamed for their children's faulty nutrition and inactivity. Very few mothers receive any nutritional guidance from their pediatrician, who doesn't know much about diet either. What is taught in medical school boils down to the usual "protein, carbohydrates and fats" doctrine, so pediatricians are unable to recognize the harm done by the children's favorite foods. **For instance, the animal products used in fast foods are heat-damaged, poorly assimilated, too high in cholesterol and salt and deficient in true nutrients—vitamins, minerals and enzymes. As a result, they don't satisfy hunger and a vicious**

cycle is created, leading to overfed but undernourished children. If a child asks for more food after a complete meal, the parent's instinctive reaction is to dish out an extra portion; they don't realize that **no additional amount of food will make up for the missing essential nutrients.**

The average American diet leaves children hungry and with low energy, so they spend a lot of their free time lounging around, doing nothing. To make up for their lethargy, they start to "look for something"; unfortunately, they find it in cola drinks containing caffeine and sugar stimulants, cigarettes full of toxic substances and eventually alcohol and street drugs, which reward them with a brief "high" and lead to addiction.

The same vicious cycle affects adults, too. Since the conventional American diet is devoid of live nutrients, the body remains unsatisfied and craves more—not quantity but quality, proper nutrition that it needs to function smoothly and well. Sadly, people don't know or understand this, and they try to satisfy their craving with rich desserts, ice cream, cakes and cookies. These don't satisfy, either, but they do create weight gain, high cholesterol, high blood pressure and eventually diabetes and worse. **Excessive weight is indeed a morbid condition, and can only be overcome by changing to a junk-free, nutrient-rich, plant-based diet.**

One doesn't need a degree in nutrition to know that all kinds of sugar are fattening and that the modern Western diet, with its vast range of convenience foods, is over-rich in sugar. However, when it comes to official policy concerning nutrition, such basic facts are often swept aside for commercial reasons, which frequently clash with the interests of public health. One such recent clash concerned the upper safe limit for sugar added to food, as recommended by the World Health Organization (WHO). Professor T. Colin Campbell[17] reported this incident in his book, *The China Study* and, with his permission, we quote his account:

> "The recommendation on added sugar is as outrageous as the one for protein. When this FNB (Food and Nutrition Board) report was being released, an expert panel put together by the

WHO (World Health Organization) and the FAO (Food and Agriculture Organization) was completing a new report on diet, nutrition and the prevention of chronic diseases. Professor Philip James was a member of this panel and a panel spokesperson on the added sugar recommendation. Early rumors of the report's findings indicated that the WHO/FAO was on the verge of recommending an upper safe limit of 10% for added sugar, far lower than the 25% established by the American FNB group. … Politics, however, had early entered the discussion, as it had done in earlier reports on added sugars. According to a news release from the director-general's office at the WHO, the US-based Sugar Association and the World Sugar Research Organization, who 'represent the interests of the sugar growers and refiners, had mounted a strong lobbying campaign in an attempt to discredit the WHO report and suppress its release.' … **According to _The Guardian_ newspaper of London, the US sugar industry was threatening to 'bring the WHO to its knees' unless it abandoned these guidelines on added sugar.** WHO people were describing the threat as 'tantamount to blackmail.' The US-based group even publicly threatened to lobby the US Congress to reduce the $406 million US funding of the WHO if it persisted in keeping the upper limit so low at 10%. There were reports … that the Bush administration was inclined to side with the sugar industry. … So, for added sugars, we now have two different upper 'safe' limits: a 10% limit for the international community and a 25% limit for the US." [Emphasis added.]

This is Professor Campbell's wry conclusion. Clearly, despite official claims, the epidemic of excessive weight hitting the American people is not solely the result of insufficient exercise!

The following is a quote from _Health Freedom News_[18]:

"Overweight Causes 100,000 Cancers Annually in the United States: According to the American Institute for Cancer Research, every year excessive weight causes more

than 100,000 cases of cancer in the United States. The Gallup-Healthways Well-being Index reported that more than 11 percent of Americans are diabetic and, given that trend, at least 15 percent of Americans will be living with diabetes by the end of 2015.

"[Being] overweight, cancer and diabetes have profound effects on quality of life and their financial cost—for individuals and the entire healthcare system—is staggering. These three conditions exemplify how lifestyle choices affect genetic expression: that is, we can activate or deactivate genes that determine why one person gets cancer or diabetes and somebody else does not. Healthcare reform without a focus on wellness does little to address why a land of plenty is so ineffective in addressing excess weight, cancer and diabetes. **As *Pulse of Health Freedom* pointed out in an article dated Oct. 20, 2009, our dollars are ill spent if we fail to champion medicine that can truly prevent and reverse conditions stemming from lifestyle choices.** On the bright side, legislation like S. 1640 (The Take Back Your Health A Cancer Therapy of 2009) does support lifestyle therapies that have significant impact on excess weight, cancer and diabetes—diseases that drain us financially while impairing quality of life." [Emphasis added.]

Joseph Mercola, MD, posted the following information in 2010[19]:

"High Fructose Corn Syrup Has Only Been Around One Generation!

"HFCS was invented in 1966 in Japan and introduced to the American market in 1975. Food and beverage manufacturers began switching their sweeteners from sucrose (table sugar) to corn syrup when they discovered that high fructose corn syrup (HFCS) was far cheaper to make—sucrose costs about three times as much as HFCS.

"HFCS is also about 20 times sweeter than table sugar. So it was expected that *less sweetener would be needed per product.* Instead, the amount of sweeteners has steadily risen.

"The switch from sugar to fructose drastically altered the average American diet. The statistics are beyond alarming:

"**• Corn syrup is now found in every type of processed, pre-packaged food you can think of. In fact, the use of HFCS in the U.S. diet increased by a whopping 10,673 percent** between 1970 and 2005, according to a report by the USDA.[1]

"• The current annual consumption of sugar is 141 pounds per person, and 63 pounds of that is HFCS.

"• Adolescents are taking in 73 grams per day of fructose, mostly from soft drinks and juice drinks—and *12 percent of their total caloric intake is from fructose alone.*

"• In the past century, fructose consumption has increased 5-fold.

"• Processed foods account for more than 90 percent of the money Americans spend on meals.

"You've probably heard the statistic that one soda a day is worth 15 pounds of fat per year. However, one soda today does not equal one soda of yesteryear. The original Coke bottle was 6.5 ounces. Now, you have 20-ounce bottles and a 44-ounce Big Gulp.

"**Tragically, many infant formulas are more than 50 percent sugar—43 percent being corn syrup solids. You might as well be giving your baby a bottle of Coke or Pepsi.**" [Emphasis added.]

CHAPTER 3 REFERENCES

1. *Taber's Cyclopedic Medical Dictionary* (Philadelphia: F. A. Davis Company, 2005), p. 1504.
2. 25 kg equals about 55 pounds.

3. Note 1 (*Taber's*, 2005), supra.

4. Ibid.

5. Definition of "morbid obesity": "Etymology: L, *morbidus*, diseased, *obesitas*, fatness an excess of body fat, or weight of 100 pounds over ideal body weight, that increases the risk of developing cardiac and endocrine disturbances, including coronary artery disease and diabetes mellitus, as well as some kinds of cancer." *Mosby's Medical Dictionary*, 8th edition. Elsevier, © 2009.

6. Note 1 (*Taber's*, 2005), supra, p. 641.

7. *Taber's Cyclopedic Medical Dictionary* (Philadelphia: F. A. Davis Company, 1993), p. 1341.

8. "Overweight and Obesity: Introduction," Centers for Disease Control and Prevention (www.cdc.gov/nccdphp/dnpa/obesity/index.htm) (page last modified: Aug. 26, 2006): "Since the mid-seventies, the prevalence of overweight and obesity has increased sharply for both adults and children. Data from two NHANES surveys show that among adults aged 20-74 years the prevalence of obesity increased from 15.0% (in the 1976-1980 survey) to 32.9% (in the 2003-2004 survey)."

9. "Obesity in children," *New England Journal of Medicine* 350 (2004): 2362-74.

10. "National diabetes fact sheet: general information and national estimates on diabetes in the United States, 2005," U.S. Department of Health and Human Services, Centers for Disease Control and Prevention (Atlanta, GA) (2005) (www.cdc.gov/diabetes/pubs/pdf/ndfs_2005.pdf).

11. "Heart Disease is the Number One Cause of Death," Centers for Disease Control and Prevention, Division for Heart Disease and Stroke Prevention (www.cdc.gov/DHDSP/announcements/american_heart_month.htm).

12. "AOA Fact Sheets: Obesity in Youth," American Obesity Association (www.obesity.org/subs/fastfacts/obesity_youth.shtml).

13. Frank Booth (boothf@missouri.edu).

14. "Research finds fatal flaw in industry's food labelling scheme" (Mar. 1, 2007), Sustainweb (www.sustainweb.org/news.php?id=169).

15. "Super Size Me," Academy Award-winning documentary film by Morgan Spurlock, director (release date: May 21, 2004) (Canada).

16. Ibid.

17. T. Colin Campbell and Thomas M. Campbell II, *The China Study: Startling Implications for Diet, Weight Loss and Long-term Health* (Dallas: BenBella Books, 2005), pp. 309-10.

18. *Health Freedom News*, Nov. 18, 2009.

19. Joseph Mercola, "This Common Food Ingredient Can Really Mess Up Your Life" [Internet]. May 15-16, 2010 [cited May 13, 2010]. Available from: www.lewrockwell.com/orig5/mercola31.1.html.

Breakdown of the Body's Defenses

The human organism evolved over millions of years as part of nature, alongside plants and animals. It was only exposed to natural substances; environment, food and shelter contained nothing artificial or alien. Our remotest ancestors enjoyed a Golden Age. Their lives were undoubtedly hard and short, but their slow evolution was totally natural and well adapted to the world in which they lived.

Changes set in with civilization, but they only became drastic and rapid after the arrival of the Industrial Revolution in the late 18th century. A second wave of even more drastic innovations followed in the developed world after World War II in the mid-20th century, changing people's daily lives, working routine, living conditions and, above all, their diet—the most important factor affecting us all. The huge development of commercial agriculture and the apparently limitless expansion of the food industry changed our "daily bread" almost beyond recognition.

However—and this is the main point—the human organism hasn't had time to adapt and adjust to these fundamental changes and therefore its defenses can't cope with the multiple challenges facing it. It fights to keep functioning normally but, undermined by polluted air, water and wrong food, it breaks down sooner or later. Unfortunately for each new generation, the breakdown now comes sooner.

Perhaps the greatest of Dr. Gerson's many revolutionary insights was his realization that the underlying causes of chronic disease were toxicity and nutritional deficiency. We will review these and some of their significant contributing factors below.

Toxicity

The air we breathe—essential to our survival—is contaminated by exhaust fumes from road traffic, tiny invisible particles that are released from tires and nestle in our lungs, residues of aircraft fuel descending from the sky and poisonous gases that countless industrial processes belch from factory chimneys or even the neighborhood dry-cleaning establishment.

Water—another necessity of life—is equally contaminated with chlorine and fluoride and residues of a wide variety of pharmaceuticals resistant to all existing purification techniques (except distillation).

Now we come to the food supply, where toxicity starts in the soil and the plants that grow on it. Highly poisonous pesticides, fungicides, herbicides and other chemicals used in commercial agriculture, often until the day of harvesting, leave residues on the plants that become our food. Many of these poisons are systemic (i.e., they permeate the produce and cannot be removed by washing). Unless we eat only organically grown foods, our daily meals are richly laced with a cocktail of agrochemicals whose cumulative effect has never been tested.

In the course of food processing, vast numbers of chemical additives are introduced, many of which are unsafe[1] . . . and worse. Their purpose is to extend shelf life (sometimes almost indefinitely), make the product look more attractive and substitute artificial flavors for the missing natural ones. "Food cosmetics," as they are ironically called, solely serve the profit-centered interests of the manufacturers and have nothing to do with healthy nutrition—on the contrary! They serve the sole purpose of enhancing manufacturers' profits. (See "Food Additives," p. 31, for the worst food additives.)

Nutritional Deficiency

Like toxicity, this disease-causing process begins in the soil. For well over 150 years, the increased use of artificial fertilizers has provided the soil with three vital minerals: nitrogen, phosphorus and potassium, disregarding the 50 or so minerals and trace elements essential to maintaining it healthy, fertile and rich in the enzymes and micro-organisms that characterize naturally fertilized, humus-rich land. As a result, it produces only deficient, nutrient-poor plants that become our equally deficient daily food.

Processing further depletes our food. All canned, jarred, boxed, smoked, pickled, bottled and otherwise conserved items are drained of their few remaining nutrients and damaged by high heat and preservatives. They lack vitamins and enzymes. The latter, vitally important for good digestion, are destroyed at a temperature of over 140° F (60° C) and can only be supplied to the body by fresh raw fruits and salads. However, few people eat enough of these to get adequate enzymes needed for a healthy system.

By now, it should be clear that the two main enemies of good health— toxicity and deficiency, which the Gerson program attempts to tackle as a first priority—add up to a single vicious cycle. **If our food were truly nutritious, our bodies would be better able to deal with toxicity, but it is not.** As a result, sooner or later the degenerative process sets in, opening the door to serious chronic disease. **Obviously, both enemies of health have to be dealt with in order to initiate healing and to restore the body's natural defenses.**

Significant Contributing Factors

Chemical Agriculture

Artificial fertilizers have been in increasing use for well over 150 years, damaging and impoverishing the soil and the microorganisms on which the health of the soil and of all plant life depends. Plants, in turn, are the food of animals and humans, and their reduced nutritional value has far-reaching effects. Dr. Gerson was one of the few visionary scientists who realized early on that there was a definite link between dietary deficiencies and diseases—and between diseases and a sick, depleted soil. He wrote, **"There is an external and an internal metabolism upon which all life depends; both are closely and inextricably connected with each other; furthermore, the reserves of both are not inexhaustible."**[2]

Once the reserves of the soil are exhausted, the plants begin to sicken. Deficient in nutrients, they lose their defenses against pests, rust, fungi and a multitude of other invaders. Hence, fungicides, pesticides and other toxic chemicals have been developed. At the beginning it was assumed that these agrochemicals were harmless if applied "as directed"; unfortunately, this has not proved to be the case.

The heavy pesticides—specifically DDT (dichloro-diphenyl-trichlo-roethane)—were first distributed halfway through World War II, around 1943. As Dr. Gerson reports in his book,[3] this and other toxic materials were found in meat, butter, milk and even mother's milk within 18 months!

Subsequently, it became clear that the toxic agrochemicals were also penetrating into the soil and the water table. These results can be seen today in several areas of California, heavily treated with huge amounts of pesticides every year, where the water and the soil are so toxic that an epidemic of primary liver cancer has hit children who played outdoors.[4]

The situation has gone from bad to worse. After DDT had been used for some time, the insect pests became resistant to it, so that heavier, even more toxic materials, such as dieldrin, had to be produced. At the same time, it transpired that the human body was *not* able to develop a resistance to those poisons. **Their effect on adults is bad enough; tragically, embryos, tiny babies and small children with their delicate constitutions suffer more serious damage to their developing bodies.**

As if dealing with the existing problems caused by agrochemicals were not enough, human health is facing the further threat posed by genetically modified (GM) food. This is an area where the conflict between powerful commercial interests and public health has come out into the open—despite the best efforts of Monsanto, a genetically modified organism (GMO) producer, to suppress data casting serious doubts on the safety of GM foods for human consumption.[5]

This is in keeping with the normal routine of agrochemical manufacturers that invariably set out to prove the safety of one or another of their products. **Anyone on an average modern diet is bound to consume the residues of several toxic substances clinging to fruits and vegetables, yet no one has ever researched the cumulative effect of this kind of toxic cocktail.**

The picture is gloomy, yet all is not lost. From small beginnings, the organic production of fruits and vegetables has grown exponentially in recent years, allowing the enlightened consumer to live on poison-free produce. **Organic food, grown on traditionally fertilized soil, has the** further advantage of containing all the minerals, trace elements, enzymes and vitamins needed for good health. This is why, in order to achieve healing, Gerson patients must use nothing but organic produce.

Enough has been said to illustrate the vicious cycle initiated by the average modern diet. Living on toxin-rich but nutrient-poor food—especially "fast food"—people begin to suffer from headaches, arthritis, insomnia, depression, frequent colds, infections, digestive problems and more. They use more over-the-counter drugs, while doctors prescribe symptom-relieving medicines that don't deal with the underlying cause of their disease.

Drugs

Half of the modern drugs could well be thrown out of the window, except that the birds might eat them.

—*Dr. M. H. Fischer, MD*

"A pill for every ill" sums up the extreme reliance on drugs that has become an integral part of today's lifestyle. One only has to turn on the television or radio to hear an endless recitation of the latest drugs being promoted to overcome every kind of human ill. **Invariably, there is also a rapidly recited and deemphasized list of the many harmful side effects of each one.**

One example of an increasingly overused drug in the public eye is Ritalin®, routinely prescribed to children suffering from so-called attention deficit hyperactivity disorder. The *Physician's Desk Reference*, which lists and describes all drugs on the market for use by physicians, specifies that it should not be used by children under the age of six years, and lists the following side effects: suppression of growth, loss of appetite, abdominal pain, weight loss, insomnia and visual disturbances.[6] (It does not mention the many documented cases[7] of suicide and unprovoked killings by youngsters on Ritalin.)

It is not hard to imagine what Ritalin and similar selective serotonin reuptake inhibitor drugs do to the child's entire developing organism and immature natural defenses. At the time of this writing, over five million American children are on Ritalin.[8] What will their state of health be like in, say, 15 years' time?

Looking at the overuse of drugs in general, the real trouble is that they only suppress symptoms and allow people to carry on with their daily routines, at least for a while. However, they never heal or clear the underlying cause of the pain or malfunction. The problem continues and gets worse; being masked by the drug, it becomes harder to diagnose. Since the body is an indivisible whole, the drug's toxicity affects not just the liver—the heart, the lungs, the kidneys and the digestive system also suffer—and the body's defenses weaken accordingly.

Food Additives

One way of healthy eating goes under the name of the "Stone Age Diet," which says, "Eat only food from which nothing has been removed, to which nothing has been added, and which would go bad if you didn't eat it immediately."[9] You would have a hard time if you tried to find such foods in any supermarket on Earth. What those temples of the food industry sell—unless they have a range of organic produce—is the exact opposite of the above rule.

The ubiquitous use of food additives, whose number is at present about 10,000,[10] serves the sole purpose of making industrially produced foods look better, taste good despite the fact that they contain inferior raw materials, have a longer shelf life and thus be more profitable. Food chemistry is so highly developed that it can mimic almost any natural flavor or scent. What it cannot do is fool the human organism into responding to these fakes as if they were the genuine article, and it only delivers chemicals of varying toxicity instead of essential nutrients.

The most widely used additives include sodium nitrite, saccharin, caffeine, olestra (a fat substitute), artificial colorings and flavorings, antioxidants, emulsifiers, flavor enhancers, thickening agents, aspartame, transfats and MSG—plus unhealthy amounts of sugar, salt and fat. They can cause a multitude of allergic reactions, such as fatigue, behavioral problems, mood swings and, after long-term use, may even lead to heart disease and cancer.

Aspartame

Aspartame deserves special scrutiny, partly because it is in approximately 6,000 food products[11] and is hard to avoid. It is now known to cause a range of serious health problems.

Among long-term regular consumers of aspartame (e.g., in Diet Coke® or as NutraSweet® in tea and coffee), it can mimic conditions such as multiple sclerosis, diabetes and its complications, arthritis, Alzheimer's disease and severe depression.[12]

These pseudo-diseases are impossible to diagnose and treat, but patients experience immediate relief if they exclude all aspartame-containing foods and drinks from their diet.[13] Since the substance is highly addictive, quitting isn't easy.

Aspartame contains methanol, a cumulative poison, which converts into formaldehyde, a known carcinogen[14]; diketopiperazine, which in animal experiments has produced brain tumors[15]; and phenylalanine, which can produce severe neurological problems.[16] It is not hard to imagine how it damages the body's defenses.

Excess Body Weight and Aspartame

Sugar consumption in the United States has been extraordinarily high.[17] People are aware that sugar is a serious cause of weight gain. Chemical manufacturers have learned how to make huge sums of money from this problem by producing artificial sweeteners that add no calories.

One such item is aspartame, known to the public as one of three items: NutraSweet®, Equal® and Spoonful®. When it was first submitted to the U.S. Food and Drug Administration (FDA), their chemists found it so seriously toxic that they would not allow it to be used in foods.[18]

After many more tests[19] plus immense political pressure and maneuvering by Donald Rumsfeld, chief executive officer of aspartame manufacturer Searle, it was finally accepted as safe by the FDA.[20] It is now found in over 6,000 food products on supermarket shelves.[21]

Aspartame is seriously toxic and has caused a severe epidemic of what mimics multiple sclerosis, but is simply aspartame poisoning.[22] Also, if exposed to temperatures above 86° F (30° C), it breaks down into methanol (wood alcohol), which is especially toxic for diabetics.[23] It can cause blindness, vertigo, stupor, abdominal pain, convulsions and kidney damage.[24]

Completely aside from these problems, aspartame is a drug that has a "contrary effect." People use "diet drinks" in the hope of consuming sweet drinks without gaining weight. The opposite is true. The Congressional Record has a notation that states, "It makes you crave carbohydrates and will make you FAT."[25]

H. J. Roberts, MD, of the Palm Beach Institute for Medical Research, diabetes specialist and world expert on aspartame, has written against the use of aspartame in his book, *Defense Against Alzheimer's Disease*. He observes that, when he got patients off aspartame, they lost an average of 19.5 pounds.[26] In his book, he also notes that aspartame poisoning is escalating Alzheimer's disease. A hospice nurse observed that some women are now being admitted with Alzheimer's at the age of 30! [27]

Dr. Louis Elias, pediatrics professor (Genetics, at Emory University) testified before Congress that, in his original lab tests, animals developed brain tumors from aspartame.[28] When Dr. [Joseph L.] Esposito was lecturing on aspartame, one physician in the audience, **a neurosurgeon, said, "When they remove brain tumors, they have found high levels of aspartame in them."**[29]

There is an excellent replacement product on the market called Stevia—a sweet food, not an additive—that actually helps the sugar metabolism and is ideal for diabetics.[30] It has now been approved as a dietary supplement by the FDA. However, for years the FDA had outlawed this sweet food because of their loyalty to Monsanto!

In 1991, the National Institutes of Health published a bibliography of 167 studies documenting the adverse effects associated with aspartame,[31] yet it is still incorporated in some 6,000 products on today's grocery shelves.[32] It is known to affect short-term memory[33] and may lead to a wide variety of diseases,[34] including:

- Migraines

- Brain tumors

- Birth defects

- Multiple sclerosis

- Alzheimer's disease

- Diabetes

- Chronic fatigue syndrome

- Epilepsy/seizures

- Fibromyalgia

Very recently, due to an enormous groundswell of resistance to the word "aspartame," Ajinomoto (its current manufacturer) has renamed it to "AminoSweet" and is marketing it as a "natural" product. We again have to urge people who want to be well or get well to always choose "organic" and fresh foods. These are as safe as possible.

Monosodium Glutamate

This flavor enhancer, developed by a Japanese food chemist in 1907, is tasteless by itself. In its original form, it was a salt derivative of a natural amino acid called "glutamate," a common substance found in every plant and animal species. **Eventually, turned into MSG, it found its way into almost every kind of convenience food—from soups, canned gravy, salad dressings, fro-** **zen/ready meals to potato chips—and into meals served in the worldwide chains of fast-food restaurants. (On food labels, it often hides behind the name "hydrolyzed vegetable protein.")**

The reason for this lavish use of MSG was discovered by John E. Erb, a research assistant at the University of Waterloo, Ontario, Canada, when he found out that laboratory mice and rats, used for studies on obese animals, had to be injected with MSG soon after birth to make them fat.[35]

Under natural circumstances, no rodents become obese; they only do so when the injected MSG triples the amount of insulin that their pancreas produces. Once fat, they are known as "MSG-treated rats."

Away from the research laboratory, MSG is added to human food for its addictive effect. As long ago as 1978, it was scientifically proven to be an addictive substance.[36] Since the food manufacturers' lobby openly states that the purpose of MSG is to make people eat more,[37] this addictive item clearly plays a major role in the current obesity epidemic.

Huge numbers of people suffer from the serious side effects of MSG, which include headaches, palpitation, vomiting, nausea, numbness, chest pain, drowsiness, facial pressure and weakness.[38] Some of these side effects are also referred to as "Chinese restaurant syndrome."

John E. Erb summed up his findings in *The Slow Poisoning of America*,[39] his book on the harmful activities of the food additive industry. Then Erb checked the cupboards in his kitchen and refrigerator and found that MSG was in everything!

A few examples are Campbell's® soups, flavored potato chips from Frito-Lay®, Nissin's Top Ramen®, Betty Crocker's Hamburger Helper®, canned gravy from Heinz®, frozen prepared meals from Swanson® and salad dressing from Kraft®. MSG is also added in abundance to the food at Burger King, McDonald's, Wendy's, Taco Bell and particularly Kentucky Fried Chicken.[40]

Although the dangers of MSG have been widely known for decades, the FDA sets no limits on how much of it may be added to foods. They claim that it is "safe" in any amount.[41]

Many people are intolerant of MSG and develop serious allergic symptoms.[42] The problem has been thoroughly studied by Jack I. Samuels and his wife, Adrilenne Samuels, PhD. Mr. Samuels is the president and co-founder of the Truth in Labeling Campaign, which was started in 1994.

The couple have worked to inform consumers, physicians, researchers and government officials of the dangers of MSG. They have testified at meetings held and/or funded by the FDA and in scientific journals.

The Samuels have warned the public that it is not easy to identify foods containing MSG due to its acceptance and long-term (grandfathered) use by the FDA.[43] **It is hidden from the public with names such as flavor enhancers, autolyzed yeast, hydrolyzed vegetable protein and textured protein. It also causes increased hunger, cravings, weight gain, water retention, irritability and fatigue.**

Here is a list of the hidden names under which MSG masquerades. These ingredients always contain processed free glutamic acid:

- Autolyzed plant protein
- Autolyzed yeast
- Autolyzed yeast extract
- Calcium caseinate
- Calcium glutamate
- Gelatin
- Glutamate
- Glutamic acid
- Anything hydrolyzed, including hydrolyzed plant protein and hydrolyzed vegetable protein
- Magnesium glutamate
- Monoammonium glutamate
- Monopotassium glutamate
- MSG
- Senomix

- Sodium caseinate
- Soy protein
- Soy protein concentrate
- Soy protein isolate
- Textured protein
- Vetsin
- Whey protein
- Whey protein concentrate
- Whey protein isolate
- Yeast extract
- Yeast food
- Yeast nutrient

These ingredients often contain or produce processed free glutamic acid:

- Barley malt
- Bouillon and broth
- Carrageenan (E407)[44]
- Citrate (E330)
- Citric acid
- Anything containing "enzymes"
- Anything "enzyme modified"
- Anything "fermented"
- Any "flavors" or "flavoring"
- Malt extract
- Maltodextrin
- Pectin (E440)

- Protease

- Anything "protein fortified"

- Seasonings

- Stock

- Soy sauce (A reader has informed us that Russell Blaylock, MD, states in his book, *Excitotoxins: The Taste That Kills*, that soy sauce *always* contains MSG.[45])

- Soy sauce extract

- Anything "ultra-pasteurized"

Here are ingredients suspected of containing or creating sufficient processed free glutamic acid that may trigger an MSG-reaction in *highly sensitive* people:

- Brown rice syrup

- Corn starch

- Corn syrup

- Dextrose

- Anything "enriched"

- Lipolyzed butter fat

- Milk powder

- Modified food starch

- Most things "low fat" or "no fat"

- Reduced fat milk (skim, 1% or 2%)

- Rice syrup

- Anything "vitamin enriched"

These work synergistically with MSG to enhance flavor. If they are present for flavoring, so is MSG:

- Disodium 5'-guanylate (E627)

- Disodium 5'-inosinate (E631)

- Disodium 5'-ribonucleotides (E635)

MSG is used by scientists to make laboratory animals fat for research purposes. Obesity will develop in these animals, even though they do not increase their food intake!

MSG appears to affect the hunger/weight control centers of the brain; however, MSG is added to so many foods that, according to the textbook, *Nutritional Biochemistry and Metabolism,* the average American consumes 1.92 pounds of MSG each year. **It is addictive and the food industry adds it to such a huge number of processed foods,[46] so that it causes people to eat more of their merchandise.**

Here is an abbreviated list of foods that contain MSG:

- Bouillon cubes

- Canned and frozen meats

- Canned soups

- Chicken stock

- Dips

- Jarred fish

- Luncheon meats

- Salad dressings

- Sauces

- Soy sauce

Altered Foods

The only way to exclude these and countless other harmful additives from one's diet is to avoid all manufactured foods. Take the more labor-intensive but health-restoring path of eating only fresh, organic natural foods, and limit restaurant meals to rare occasions.

Additive-filled junk food not only harms the body but is also a powerful trigger for antisocial behavior. Researchers both in California and in

England have run experiments in prisons housing young male criminals, giving them supplements containing vitamins, minerals and essential fatty acids over several months, and monitoring their behavior. In both countries, minor offenses dropped by 33%; serious ones, including violence, dropped by 37% to 38%.[47] Take those findings out of the prison setting and it becomes obvious that much antisocial behavior in society can be ascribed directly to harmful toxic food additives—yet another powerful argument for avoiding junk food of all kinds.

Transfats

Described variously as the world's unhealthiest food and/or as "heart attack in a box," these ubiquitous food components are produced by hydrogenating vegetable oil to turn a liquid into a solid substance. Transfats or hydrogenated vegetable oils (HVOs) are known to increase the levels of LDL (low-density lipoprotein) or "bad cholesterol," while reducing those of HDL (high-density lipoprotein), the "good" variety. They leave fatty deposits in the arteries, cause digestive disorders and reduce the absorption rate of essential vitamins and minerals.

The Harvard School of Public Health has estimated that at least 30,000 people—probably 100,000—die every year in the United States from cardiovascular disease, caused by eating HVOs found in most convenience foods.[48] The American nutritionist, Mary Enig, has stated that transfats disrupt the cellular function of the body, weakening its power to expel wastes and toxins.[49] This opens the door to heart disease, diabetes, cancer, poor immunity and obesity.

The good news is that, since January 2006, under U.S. government regulations, food manufacturers must state the amount of transfats contained in their products.[50] Some have already started to remove transfats from their output. The British Soil Association, flagship of the organic movement in the United Kingdom, has recently declared that all additives, including transfats, MSG and aspartame, are absolutely banned from all organic products[51]—yet another reason to commit ourselves to organic food.

Salt and Sodium

The dangers of food additives should not blind us to the fact that the first major culprit of the average modern diet is salt (sodium)—the very substance that's hardest to avoid. Despite official warnings against its overuse,[52] salt consumption in the Western world is alarmingly high. Within the body, it causes water retention, leading to edema and weight gain. **Salt also puts an unreasonable burden on the kidneys, raises blood pressure, deadens the taste buds so that more and more is needed to produce an effect and interferes with the digestive process.**

People are so used to adding salt to their food that they find it difficult to eat anything unsalted! This is understandable since almost all the food is grown in deficient soil and then boiled in lots of water. When the water is thrown out, the flavor goes with it, as well as any remaining food value.

In spite of repeated warnings about the danger of using salt, its consumption is extremely high—even higher in the United States than in European countries.[53]

Salt forces the body to retain water, which it uses to dilute the toxic effect of sodium in the cells. This results in edema of the tissues. Salt damages the kidneys and the digestive process, so the body is unable to readily absorb calcium.[54]

Most people are not aware that such disturbances cause the body to be unable to use foods, which then act as toxins (poisons). Toxins are also defined as "enzyme inhibitors," further interfering with normal metabolism. It is important to understand that, among other activities, kidneys are involved in excreting the end products of protein digestion and sodium; in other words, they are very important detoxifying organs. Therefore, with poor kidney function, these end products are not adequately excreted and cause a great deal of toxicity, pain and "inflammation."[55]

The dangers of food additives should not blind us to the fact that the first major culprit of the average modern diet is salt (sodium)—the very substance that's the hardest to avoid. Despite official warnings against its overuse,[56] salt consumption in the Western world is alarmingly high. Within the body, it causes water retention, leading to edema and weight gain. Salt also puts an unreasonable burden on the kidneys, raises blood pressure, deadens the taste buds so that more and more is needed to produce an effect and interferes with the digestive process.

Animal Protein

Since meat is a valued staple item of the modern diet, it may sound surprising that excess animal proteins behave as toxins in the body. The fact is that the human organism, with its long intestinal tract, is not designed to cope with a diet high in animal proteins. (By contrast, the intestinal tract of carnivores, such as lions and other big cats, is short—hence the waste products of the digested meat are eliminated quickly.) The ideal diet for humans should be predominantly plant based, with a minimum of animal proteins[57]; today the opposite applies.

As we go through life, we become less able to digest animal proteins. These poorly digested, incompletely broken-down parts linger in the body as toxins. The animal fats contained in almost all meat, poultry and dairy produce are also digested inadequately as the body ages and its enzymes no longer function efficiently. **It is also important to note that food animals are raised on unhealthy food treated with hormones, antibiotics and synthetic growth promoters. Whatever they are forced**

to consume remains in the meat, eggs and milk products that finally land on our tables, adding to the already heavy toxic load we are unwittingly carrying.

The body attempts to get rid of all these harmful substances to protect itself; unfortunately, in addition to the massive burden of toxins with which it needs to deal, it also confronts the problem of deficiency.

Fluoride

Among the factors undermining the body's defenses, fluoride deserves special attention. While exorbitant dental health claims are made for it by commercial interests, **it is in fact a dangerous poison, an industrial waste containing small amounts of lead, mercury, beryllium and arsenic.**[58] The official reason why the U.S. government promotes the compulsory addition of fluoride to drinking water is to improve children's dental health, which, as common sense recognizes, is not undermined by a shortage of fluoride but by an unhealthy diet, insufficient dental hygiene and too many sweets.

According to some experts,[59] **fluoride only protects the teeth of children up to the age of five.** Since that age group comprises only a small percentage of the population, it seems indefensible to force this highly controversial chemical onto everybody, irrespective of their age and dental condition.

Moreover, there is evidence[60] to show that fluoridation does not lastingly improve children's dental health. On the other hand, it causes fluorosis in one of every eight children, resulting in mottled, discolored teeth.[61] In the United States, according to figures released in 2003, despite fluoridation, more than half of children aged six to eight years and two-thirds of all 15-year-olds suffer from dental decay.[62] **It is also claimed that the prolonged intake of fluoride can be linked to increased risk of cancers, hip fractures, osteoporosis, kidney trouble and even birth defects.**[63]

The late Dean Burk, MD, who had worked for more than 30 years as chief chemist at the U.S. National Cancer Institute (NCI), declared, "Fluoride causes more human cancer death, and causes it faster, than

any other chemical."[64] Following a 17-year study, the NCI found that, as fluoridation increased, so did oral cancer and osteosarcoma, a rare form of bone cancer, in young men.[65]

Despite the NCI study's conclusions, the pro-fluoride camp is doing its utmost to hide and deny the harmful effects of the chemical. One such attempt led to an uproar among scientists in 2006, when it transpired that Professor Chester Douglass of the Harvard Dental School had kept secret the findings of his graduate student Elise B. Bassin for four years. In her 2001 thesis, Bassin discussed the association between fluoride and cancer, particularly osteosarcoma—bone cancer—in young males. When her findings were finally published in May 2006, and the truth came out to general consternation among researchers, **Harvard exonerated Professor Douglass from any wrongdoing and conflict of interest, although he is widely known to be a paid consultant for the toothpaste industry, which is a major user of fluoride.**[66]

Up to 500 letters of protest have been sent to Harvard's President Bok, among them a blistering one from Professor Samuel Epstein, Chairman of the Cancer Prevention Coalition, demanding "a full and watertight explanation of this extraordinary action."[67] At the time of this writing, Professor Douglass is said to have contributed $1 million to the new dentistry building of Harvard—and his crime has thus been "forgiven."

This story is just one of many examples showing how assiduously vested interests fight to protect their profitable products, even at the risk of endangering public health.

Nicotine and Alcohol

The health ravages caused by smoking have been widely known for a long time, yet the habit persists. Smokers use cigarettes either as a stimulant or as an aid to relaxation. In either case, the desired effect wears off quickly and has to be renewed, hence the self-destructive routine of chain smoking.

The main active ingredient of tobacco is nicotine, authoritatively described as "one of the most toxic and addictive of all poisons"[68] yet nicotine is not the only toxic product of smoking. The tars produced by the burning process line the lungs and eventually cause emphysema and cancer.[69]

Smokers tend to assume that they are only damaging their lungs; however, the poisons contained in cigarettes pervade the entire organism, damaging all organs. Bladder cancer, for instance, occurs more frequently among smokers than abstainers.[70] There is also the detrimental effect of the well-documented "second-hand smoke" on the smoker's family and workmates.[71] What may appear to many—even today—as an acceptable social habit is in fact a serious attack on our natural defenses.

The same applies to alcohol, which ideally should only be consumed occasionally and in small amounts. If consumed in excess, alcohol can lead to chronic alcoholism. It is poisonous to the brain and even more so to the liver, and can cause gastritis, pancreatitis, seizures and delirium. In extreme cases, it leads to cirrhosis of the liver and death.[72] Since the liver is a key organ, it is easy to see how its destruction by uncontrolled drinking undermines the entire organism.

We have shown only a few of the aggressively toxic and damaging factors that lead to disease. **If toxicity and deficiency are, as Dr. Gerson maintained, the two major causes of degenerative problems, they are necessarily the two main areas needing to be addressed for healing. If the body is sick due to toxicity and deficiency, in order to heal, one must *detoxify* as well as *intensively restore nutrients.***

While food is deficient, it is further depleted by processing. All canned, jarred, boxed, preserved, bottled and otherwise prepared items are damaged by high heat and preservatives, and contain little nutrition. **If our food were truly nutritious, our bodies would be better able to deal with toxicity, but it is not. As a result, the degenerative process sets in, opening the door to serious chronic disease.**

Processed foods are also depleted of vitamins and enzymes.[73] Enzymes are destroyed at a temperature of 140° F[74] and can only be supplied to the body via raw food such as fruit and raw salads and their fresh juices. Few people consume enough of these to supply adequate quantities of enzymes and vitamins for a healthy system.

It is clear that the above problems have to be dealt with in order to initiate healing.

CHAPTER 4 REFERENCES

1. Sally Fallon, "Dirty Secrets of the Food Processing Industry," presentation given at the annual conference of Consumer Health of Canada (March 2002) (www.westonaprice.org/modernfood/dirty-secrets.html).

2. M. Gerson, *A Cancer Therapy: Results of Fifty Cases and The Cure of Advanced Cancer by Diet Therapy: A Summary of Thirty Years of Clinical Experimentation,* 6th ed. (San Diego, CA: Gerson Institute, 1999).

3. Ibid., pp. 145-173.

4. B. P. Baker, Charles M. Benbrook, E. Groth III and K. Lutz Benbrook, "Pesticide residues in conventional, integrated pest management (IPM)-grown and organic foods: insights from three US data sets," Taylor and Francis Ltd., *Food Additives and Contaminants* 19 (5) (May 2002): 427-446(20).

5. G. Lean, "Revealed: health fears over secret study into GM food," *The Independent on Sunday* (London) (May 22, 2005).

6. PDR Drug information for RITALIN® HYDROCHLORIDE (Novartis) (methylphenidate hydrochloride) tablets USP RITALIN-SR® (methylphenidate hydrochloride) USP sustained-release tablets (www.ritalindeath.com/Ritalin-PDR.htm).

7. "Learning and Learning Disabilities: Ritalin Side Effects," Audiblox (www.audiblox2000.com/learning_disabilities/ritalin.htm).

8. "Every day five million children in America line up for their daily dose of Ritalin." (www.add-adhd-help-center.com/ritalin_side_effects.htm). "More than 8 million children and teenagers are prescribed psychiatric drugs: antidepressants, stimulants and antipsychotics." (www.scribd.com/doc/7432784/Anti-Depressants-Adderall-Bi-Polar-Anxiety-Disorder-ADHD-Ritalin-Your-Childs-Future). "Ritalin: Keeping Kids Cool and in School" ("There are currently an estimated 5 million school-age children on the drug. Another 2 million children are thought to be on other psychiatric

drugs, such as Adderall and Dexedrine. Production of these drugs has grown 2000%, according to the Drug Enforcement Agency.") (http://social.jrank.org/pages/1011/Special-Needs-Gifts-Issues-Ritalin-Keeping-Kids-Cool-in-School.html).

9. Richard Mackarness, *Eat Fat and Grow Slim* (London: Harvill Press, 1958; London: Fontana/Collins, revised and extended edition, 1975).

10. Pat Thomas, in "What's in this Stuff?," reports that "more than 10,000 chemicals are added to food these days." (www.informationliberation.com/?id=21399).

11. The Nutrasweet Co. (www.nutrasweet.com).

12. "… a few of the published associations in aspartame reactors. They include the initiation or aggravation of diabetes mellitus, hypoglycemia, convulsions, headache, depression, other psychiatric states, hyperthyroidism, hypertension and arthritis; the simulation of multiple sclerosis, Alzheimer's disease and lupus erythematosus; increasing aspartame addiction[12]; an apparent causative role in brain tumors[10]; a neurologic condition in overweight young women known as pseudotumor cerebri; and even the carpal tunnel syndrome.[11]" (www.wnho.net/fdaapprovedepidemic.htm) H. J. Roberts, "Aspartame (NutraSweet) addiction." *Townsend Letter for Doctors & Patients* 2000; 198 (January): 52-57.

13. www.holisticmed.com/aspartame/adverse.txt.

14. Betty Martini, MD, "Aspartame: No Hoax, Crime of the Century (Front Groups in Violation of Title 18, Section 1001 When They Lie About the Aspartame Issue and Stumble Others)" (Duluth, GA), Mission Possible International (Jul. 18, 2004) (www.wnho.net/aspartame_no_hoax.htm).

15. Louis Elsas testifies before Congress. Animals developed brain tumors; *see also* Note 14 (Martini), supra.

16. Ibid.

17. T. Colin Campbell and Thomas M. Campbell II, *The China Study: Startling Implications for Diet, Weight Loss and Long-term Health* (Dallas: BenBella Books, 2005), p. 98.

18. "Aspartame, Decision of the Public Board of Inquiry" (Sept. 30, 1980), Department of Health and Human Services, Food and Drug Administration [Docket number 75F-0355] (www.sweetpoison.com/_articles/pdfs/fdapetition.pdf).

19. Aspartame Toxicity Information Center (www.holisticmed.com/aspartame/adverse.txt).

20. James Turner, ESQ, Director of the National Institute of Science, Law, and Public Policy (NISLAPP), *Aspartame/NutraSweet: The History of the Aspartame Controversy* (Washington, DC: National Institute of Science, Law, and Public Policy).

21. FoodFacts.com: "It is now estimated that over 6,000 food and drink products worldwide contain this popular artificial sweetener." (blog.foodfacts.com/index.php/2009/09/08/aspartame-nutrition-facts). The Aspartame Information Center quotes 6,000 products as containing aspartame (www.aspartame.org/aspartame_products.html).

22. www.fda.gov/ohrms/dockets/DOCKETS/02p0317/02P-0317_emc-000429-01.pdf (page 2 of 18).

23. www.dorway.com/betty/diabetes.html.

24. H. J. Roberts, *Aspartame Disease: An Ignored Epidemic* (W. Palm Beach, FL: Sunshine Sentinel Press, 2001). A table in this publication identifies "blindness," "kidney stones," "convulsions" and "grand mal" attacks as symptoms of aspartame poisoning.

25. Congressional Record, Senate, S-5511, May 7, 1985, and part of the protest of the National Soft Drink Association, now American Beverage, is this statement: "Aspartame has been demonstrated to inhibit the carbohydrate-induced synthesis of the neurotransmitter serotonin (Wurtman affidavit). Serotonin blunts the sensation of craving carbohydrates and this is part of the body's feedback system that helps limit consumption of carbohydrate to appropriate levels. Its inhibition by aspartame could lead to the anomalous result of a diet product causing increased consumption of carbohydrates."

26. H. J. Roberts, MD, *Defense Against Alzheimer's Disease* (W. Palm Beach, FL: Sunshine Sentinel Press, April 1995).

27. Ibid.

28. Mary Nash Stoddard, *Deadly Deception: Story of Aspartame: Shocking Expose of the World's Most Controversial Sweetener* (Dallas: Odenwald Press, August 1998). This book also contains the full story and timeline of the campaign to get aspartame approved by the FDA, despite its known dangers. Michael Barbee, *Politically Incorrect Nutrition: Finding Reality in the Mire of Food Industry Propaganda* (Ridgefield, CT: Vital Health Publishing, April 2004). In this book, Barbee quotes Dr. Louis Elias, Pediatric Professor in Genetics at Emory University.

29. A resident of Marietta, Georgia, "Dr. Joe" is the president of Health Plus Wellness Center, a multidisciplinary health care center specializing in preventive health care and life extension. He is also the author of *Eating Right* (www.rense.com/health/sweetners.htm).

30. D. Gates, "The FDA and Stevia"; [Internet]. Bogart (GA): Body Ecology; 2010 [cited May 15, 2010]. Available from: www.stevia.net/fda.htm. Note: the Stevia site is part of the Body Ecology site (www.bodyecology.com). FDA statement that there is no basis to object to the use of certain refined Stevia preparations: www.fda.gov/AboutFDA/Basics/ucm194320.htm. Stevia Import Alert from FDA site: www.accessdata.fda.gov/cms_ia/ importalert_119.html.

31. U.S. National Institutes of Health, "Adverse Effects of Aspartame: January '86 through December '90" (1991), a bibliography of 167 studies documenting adverse effects associated with aspartame.

32. Note 21 (aspartame), supra.

33. www.dorway.com/92symptomsfotocopy.html.

34. Ibid.

35. John E. and T. M. Erb, *The Slow Poisoning of America* (available on-line at https://www.spofamerica.com).

36. Ibid.

37. Ibid.

38. www.dorway.com/92symptomsfotocopy.html.

39. Note 35 (Erb), supra.

40. Burger King (www.bk.com/cms/en/us/cms_out/digital_assets/files/pages/ IngredientsDeclaration.pdf); McDonald's (nutrition.mcdonalds.com/ nutritionexchange/ingredientslist.pdf); Wendy's (http://wendys.com/food/ pdf/us/nutrition.pdf); Taco Bell (www.tacobell.com/nutrition/ingredient-statement); Kentucky Fried Chicken (www.kfc.com/nutrition/pdf/ kfc_ingredients_may10.pdf).

41. As quoted from herbsspices, Monday (4/12/2010), the U.S. Food and Drug Administration (FDA) acknowledge MSG as safe a product as salt, pepper and sugar (http://medicmagic.net/how-safe-is-msg-to-consume.html#more-4049).

42. www.truthinlabeling.org/I.AreYouSensitive.html.

43. www.truthinlabeling.com/SomethingToThinkAbout.html.

44. This appears to be the EU food additive "E number" or classification. From Wikipedia.com: "When used in food products, carrageenan has the EU additive E-number E407 or E407a when present as 'processed eucheuma seaweed,' and is commonly used as an emulsifier." From *The Free Dictionary*: "citric acid n: chemistry / Elements & Compounds) a water-soluble weak tribasic acid found in many fruits, esp citrus fruits, and used in pharmaceuticals and as a flavouring (E330)."

45. Russell Blaylock, MD, *Excitotoxins: The Taste That Kills* (Albuquerque: Health Press, 1997), p. xx.

46. www.ncbi.nlm.nih.gov/pubmed/3785512?dopt=Abstract&holding=npg. "Q: What is MSG and what is the problem with it? A: MSG stands for monosodium glutamate, a substance extracted from grains or beets. In the Eastern world it is referred to as the 'magic powder of the East.' We won't bore you with it's [sic] chemical properties. There is great variation in how much MSG can be found in foods, but according to the textbook— NUTRITIONAL BIOCHEMISTRY AND METABOLISM—the average American consumes 1.92 pounds of MSG each year." (www.carbohydrateaddicts.com/msg.html).

47. B. Gesch, London press conference, Royal College of Psychiatrists (Jun. 25, 2002); S. Schoenthaler, *Anti-Ageing Medical Publications,* Vol. III. (Marina del Rey, CA: Health Quest Publications, 1999).

48. D. Mozaffarian, et al., "Trans Fatty Acids and Cardiovascular Disease," *New England Journal of Medicine* 15 (354) (Apr. 13, 2006): 1601-1613; *see also* "Trans Fatty Acids and Coronary Heart Disease" ("In an updated analysis of the trans fat-heart disease link, HSPH researchers have found that removing trans fats from the industrial food supply could prevent tens of thousands of heart attacks and cardiac deaths each year in the U.S. The findings are published in the April 13, 2006 issue of the New England Journal of Medicine. . . . Trans fats have also been associated with an increased risk of coronary heart disease in epidemiologic studies. . . . Based on the available metabolic studies, we estimated in a 1994 report that approximately 30,000 premature coronary heart disease deaths annually could be attributable to consumption of trans fatty acids.[4]" Note 4: W. C. Willett, A. Ascherio, "Trans fatty acids: Are the effects only marginal?," *Am J Public Health* 1994; 84: 722-724.) (www.hsph.harvard.edu/reviews/transfats.html)

49. Interview with Richard A. Passwater, "Health Risks from Processed Foods and the Dangers of Trans Fats."

50. "Food Labeling: Trans Fatty Acids in Nutrition Labeling . . ." U.S. Department of Health and Human Services, FDA 21 CFR Part 101, Federal Register (Jul. 11, 2003), p. 41434.

51. "What we can say—the quality and benefits of organic food," British Soil Association information sheet, Version 4 (Nov. 24, 2005).

52. "Excessive Sodium is One of the Greatest Health Threats in Foods," World Health Organization (WHO) report from October 2006 meeting in Paris,

part of the implementation of the WHO's Global Strategy on Diet, Physical Activity and Health.

53. Lawrence J. Appel, MD, MPH. and Cheryl A. M. Anderson, PhD, MPH, "Compelling Evidence for Public Health Action to Reduce Salt Intake," *New England Journal of Medicine* editorial (10.1056/nejme0910352 nejm.org); "Addressing salt intakes in Europe," FOOD TODAY European Food Information Council, August 2010 (www.eufic.org/article/en/artid/addressing-salt-intakes-in-Europe).

54. C. Gerson and B. Bishop, *Healing the Gerson Way: Defeating Cancer and Other Chronic Diseases*, Second Edition (Carmel, CA: Totality Books, 2009), p. 18.

55. *Taber's Cyclopedic Medical Dictionary*, 20th edition (Philadelphia: F. A. Davis Company, 2005), p. 1175.

56. Note 17 (Campbell), supra.

57. Emma Young, "Trace arsenic in water raises cancer risk," *New Scientist* (Sept. 14, 2001).

58. J. A. Brunette and J. P. Carlos, "Recent Trends in Dental Caries in U.S. Children and the Effect of Water Fluoridation," *Journal of Dental Research* 69 (Spec. Issue February 1990): 723-727.

59. Ibid.

60. M. A. Awad, J. A. Hargreaves, and G. W. Thompson, "Dental Caries and Fluorosis in 7-9 and 11-14 Year Old Children Who Received Fluoride Supplements from Birth," *Journal of the Canadian Dental Association* 60 (4) (1991): 318-322.

61. C. H. Shiboski, et al., "The association of early childhood caries and race/ethnicity among California preschool children," *Journal of Public Health Dentistry* 63 (1) (2003): 38-46.

62. Elise B. Bassin, D. Wypij, R. B. Davis and M. A. Mittleman, "Age-specific fluoride exposure in drinking water and osteosarcoma (United States)," *Cancer Causes and Control* 17 (2006): 421-428.

63. Dean Burk, MD, Congressional Record (Jul. 21, 1976).

64. Perry D. Cohn, "A Brief Report on the Association of Drinking Water Fluoridation and the Incidence of Osteosarcoma Among Young Males," Environmental Health Service, New Jersey Department of Health (Nov. 8, 1992). In 1992, the New Jersey State Department of Health released the results of a study which found six times more bone cancer among males under the age of 20 living in communities with fluoridated water.

65. Juliet Eilperin, "Professor at Harvard Is Being Investigated, Fluoride-Cancer Link May Have Been Hidden," *The Washington Post* (Jul. 13, 2005), p. A03.

66. Letter from Professor Samuel Epstein to Harvard University President Derek C. Bok (Aug. 31, 2006).

67. Note 55 (*Taber's*), p. 1468.

68. "Questions About Smoking, Tobacco, and Health," American Cancer Society (www.cancer.org/docroot/PED/content/PED_10_2x_Questions_About_Smoking_Tobacco_and_Health.asp).

69. "Detailed Guide: Bladder Cancer, What Are the Risk Factors for Bladder Cancer,?" American Cancer Society (www.cancer.org/docroot/cri/content/cri_2_4_2x_what_are_the_risk_factors_for_bladder_cancer_44.asp).

70. "Secondhand Smoke—It Takes Your Breath Away: Secondhand Smoke is unhealthy . . ." New York State Department of Health (www.health.state.ny.us/prevention/tobacco_control/second/second.htm).

72. Howard J. Worman, MD, "Alcoholic Liver Disease," Columbia University Department of Medicine (http://cpmcnet.columbia.edu/dept/gi/alcohol.html).

73. Natural Health Restored, "Refined Foods And Processed Foods" (www.natural-health-restored.com/refined-foods.html).

74. "Why is an enzyme destroyed by high temperature?" (http://answers.yahoo.com/question/index?qid=20070704113453AAmUvem).

CHAPTER 5

Diabetes: A Disease of Modern Civilization

It is an astonishing fact of the 21st century that, instead of enjoying good health and fitness, so many people in the developed world suffer from a multitude of complaints and diseases that a few generations ago were much less widespread. Worse still, these conditions are no longer limited to the middle-aged and elderly but instead attack ever-younger generations. Because of their comparative novelty, they are often called "diseases of modern civilization."

This sounds like a kind of justification, as if they were the price we have to pay for our unprecedented degree of technological development, comfort and consumer choice; in other words, they are a direct consequence of today's denatured, overcivilized lifestyle. Whether or not that is so, orthodox medicine deems these diseases incurable. All it can offer is symptomatic treatment, which only works up to a point and for a limited time, and has serious side effects.

What exactly is it in modern civilization that can be blamed for the deterioration of public health? The accepted culprits are widespread pollution of air, water and soil; the consequences of climate change; vastly increased levels of noise, violence and general insecurity; social tensions; stress; and the breakdown of law and order in many areas of life. All of this is true and valid. Oddly enough, the one overwhelming factor that affects every living person is not included in the list of harmful influences, namely the huge dietary changes that have taken place in the developed world over the past century or so.

This is amazing if we consider that the quality of the food and drink we consume every day of our lives is bound to have a powerful effect on our state of health. It becomes less surprising if we remember that the science of nutrition is conspicuously absent from the training of doctors. The resulting ignorance deprives them of a powerful yet gentle method of healing that is able to turn officially incurable conditions into curable ones. One can only hope that, at some time in the future, this method will enter mainstream medicine.

Diabetes

Diabetes is the #6 disease killer of Americans, following heart and circulatory disease and cancer.[1] We need to distinguish between two different types of the disease—juvenile diabetes (type 1) and age-onset diabetes (type 2)—and each requires a different approach, as described below.

About 1% of insulin-dependent diabetes is considered "brittle" or "labile" diabetes. Often the lack of control has to do with, or is caused by, psychological or stress-related factors, leading to failure by the patient to take the prescribed insulin medication.

Generally speaking, it's fair to say that "the usual suspect," namely the modern American diet with its excessively high sugar and fat content, is largely to blame for the exponential rise in cases of diabetes. **If you add up all the sugar that an average American adult consumes daily in the form of sweets, cookies, cakes, convenience foods, ice cream and the worst culprit—soft drinks—the sum total is pretty frightening.** The human body and its most concerned organ, the pancreas, are unable to deal with this onslaught. After a while, diabetes sets in; however, the causation of juvenile diabetes is a different story.

Juvenile diabetes is described as "insulin dependent,"[2] which is correct, since those suffering from it do not produce enough insulin to satisfy their bodies' needs. Insulin is a hormone, secreted by the Islets of Langerhans in the pancreas. It is essential for the proper metabolism of blood sugar and for the maintenance of proper blood sugar level. Insufficient production of insulin is generally due to severe damage to, or infection of, the pancreas, which leads to the Islets of Langerhans being damaged or partly destroyed. The remaining ones are unable to produce enough insulin.

In many cases, the problem starts in early childhood, hence the name "juvenile." Children tend to catch colds and flu fairly often, and their concerned parents take them to a pediatrician who routinely prescribes antibiotics. These suppress and temporarily clear the symptoms but tend to damage the children's immune system. As a result, more infections develop until at some stage the apparent flu is very severe, persists for some weeks and finally slowly clears. That flu turns out to have been pancreatitis (i.e., inflammation of the pancreas). A short time later, the child is diagnosed with diabetes.

In this case, not enough natural insulin is produced, and the child becomes insulin dependent and must be injected daily with the missing hormone. Sadly, the problem is lifelong and worsens over time. Since the patient is advised to eat a largely protein-based diet, excluding carbohydrates, eventually the kidneys are affected, leading to the need for kidney dialysis. Further difficulties arise, including plaque formation and circulatory problems, and even loss of toes, feet or legs, due to insufficient circulation and resulting gangrene. During adolescence, such children are not able to concentrate or do well in their studies nor do they grow at the same rate as their peers.

These multiple problems arising at a young age have been relieved by the Gerson Therapy. Obviously, the treatment has to be modified to suit the special needs of the patients: They are given less carrot and apple juice and more green leaf juice. Potatoes are cut out in favor of vegetables and raw foods, and little fruit is given, mainly apples and melons. We have observed that most patients on the Gerson Therapy are eventually able to cut down considerably on the dosage used.

One 12-year-old boy was able to decrease his insulin requirement by two-thirds of the original dose. He became an "A" student and even caught up with his classmates' growth. In other words, his condition had greatly improved; however, he could not be cured (i.e., totally freed from his need for insulin) for it was impossible to restore the destroyed Islets of Langerhans, which should have produced the necessary natural insulin. This boy's Gerson medication was augmented by chromium picolinate to boost his insulin output, but it did not come back to normal.

Caution: **Once a patient has been started on dialysis, *the Gerson Therapy cannot be used.***

Age-onset diabetes can be solved with the Gerson Therapy. Patients suffering from this condition actually produce an adequate amount of insulin. The problem is that this insulin is unable to reach the relevant receptors within the cells for these are blocked by excess cholesterol.[3]

As far as the majority of diabetes patients are concerned, they benefit from the Gerson program which, with its exclusion of animal products, is free from cholesterol. More importantly, the restored enzyme activity, together with the high omega-3 content of the flaxseed oil, is able to clear the cholesterol from the body tissues.

In most patients, excess cholesterol gets cleared out within a week or two, even though they no longer take their cholesterol-lowering drugs. It takes only a short time before the available natural insulin reaches its destination in the cells; the excess glucose (sugar) in the bloodstream is reduced to normal so there is no further need for additional insulin.

These patients are also restricted at the start of the therapy in their intake of carrot and apple juice and sweet fruit, but they can before long embark on a regular Gerson Therapy with the usual juices, potato-rich meals and oatmeal with fruit for breakfast. They, too, are supplemented with chromium picolinate but can drop this provided their blood sugar remains normal.

Age-onset Diabetes Protocol

A majority of people suffering from age-onset diabetes are found to actually produce adequate levels of insulin. In other words, this disease is not caused by a lack or an insufficient amount of insulin.

Keeping in mind what has been said about age-onset diabetes being a problem of excess cholesterol blocking the insulin receptors in the cell, the Gerson Therapy is a powerful way to overcome the problem because it includes the following benefits:

- It is totally devoid of cholesterol (animal fats).
- It is capable of dissolving and reducing cholesterol deposits.
- It allows the available insulin to reach the insulin receptors within each cell.

If a patient is on insulin, it is unwise to discontinue it immediately. As the Gerson Therapy becomes effective (generally within a week), insulin can be reduced in conjunction with blood analyses.

For those who are not on insulin, the therapy is used at a somewhat modified level for the first two to three weeks:

- The patient uses less stewed fruit or raw fruit sources for the breakfast oatmeal.

- In severe cases, the oatmeal has to be omitted for the first few days; raw salads and Hippocrates soup, for example, have to be served for breakfast.

- The number of apple/carrot juices is reduced, and those juices are replaced by the green juices (Chapter 11, "Preparing Food and Juices—The Basic Rules," p. 103). For example, instead of the usual five 8-ounce glasses of apple/carrot juice, use only three and replace the two omitted glasses with green juice. Instead of orange juice at breakfast, use grapefruit juice, which contains less sugar. Add to the usual Gerson supplements 3 capsules/day of chromium picolinate (200 mcg per capsule), which can be discontinued, usually within a week or two, when blood sugar remains stable.

- Omit bananas, dried fruit, grapes and other very sweet fruit. Instead, use apples, pears, cherries in season, plums and melons.

As blood sugar reaches a normal level, return to apple/carrot juices and the regular Gerson Therapy, including oatmeal with raw or stewed fruit for breakfast and orange juice. Avoid dried fruit and bananas for a longer period of time.

Case History

Our most severely ill diabetic patient was a 41-year-old man weighing over 300 pounds. His blood sugar ran over 340 (normal is below 120) and was uncontrollable with insulin and/or other medications. He had had a heart attack at age 38 and was left with a dangerously high blood pressure of 240/110 (normal is 120/80), also uncontrolled by drugs. He suffered from gout as well. If he had omitted his gout medication for a single day, he would have had to endure an excruciatingly painful attack.

On the Gerson Therapy, he was eating mainly vegetables and raw salads with green juices, and his diet was restricted to one potato a day. Instead of oatmeal in the morning, he received a plateful of mixed raw vegetables. He also used the usual enemas and took chromium picolinate along with the other Gerson medication. Insulin had to be continued at the start of the treatment as needed, the requirement being checked by regular blood tests.

The patient lost between one and two pounds a day without ever being hungry. On top of his three regular meals, he was given a plate of raw vegetables for snacks in his room. (Nondiabetic patients receive a fruit plate to eat as snacks during the night or between meals should they feel hungry.) His vegetable plate contained carrot and celery strips, tomatoes, cauliflower florets and radishes. His gout medication was discontinued immediately after starting the treatment without bringing on an attack.

At the end of 10 weeks, the patient's blood sugar was normal and he was able to discontinue the insulin injections. His weight had come down by almost 100 pounds, and at 6'2" he weighed an almost normal 210 pounds. Finally, his blood pressure had also dropped to a normal level without the need for drugs.

Confronting Chronic Conditions

As various serious diseases have silently crept up on us, becoming part of our way of life—and death—we tend to take them for granted and no longer question their growing prevalence or why they cut short the lives of so many people in their prime. **Clearly the chronic, incurable diseases inflicted on us are due to the faulty, health-destroying dietary habits of modern civilization. Nowadays, people truly dig their graves with their teeth, not realizing the harm they are doing to themselves.**

Now is the moment to ask questions, listen to the answers and change our lives for the better. **The good news is that the severe health damage caused by the wrong diet can be undone by the right one.** This applies as much to the killer diseases we have reviewed as to the many chronic degenerative conditions that can drag on for many years, causing much pain, discomfort, depression and poor quality of life. Modern medicine can ease the pain with allopathic drugs but is unable to eliminate the basic problem. **Indeed, many people believe that their diabetes is incurable, but they are wrong.**

Assorted Enemies of Health

Although this book focuses on diabetes, there are more than 1,500 different conditions and complaints that blight the lives of vast numbers of people in the developed world. These represent only a tiny part of the grand total of chronic conditions that are erroneously accepted as inevitable and incurable. Despite their surprisingly varied nature, **these enemies of health have one thing in common: They originate in faulty nutrition and therefore respond positively to the Gerson protocol.**

An Afterthought

There are some conditions that do not qualify as killer diseases, yet they insidiously undermine the organism over a long time and eventually contribute to a major health breakdown. Prior to that, they also cause much pain and discomfort, but these are easily repressed or at least eased with allopathic drugs, enabling sufferers to lead a normal life. As a result, people either don't take their problem (e.g., dental health) sufficiently seriously, or they believe that their pain or disease is incurable and therefore nothing can be done about it.

Take heart! You have heard that "chronic disease," including diabetes, is "incurable," but clinical evidence has shown that the Gerson Therapy can reverse almost all diseases considered chronic. The experience of thousands of patients over the best part of the past century has demonstrated the therapy's power to substantially improve the quality of life for type 1 diabetics, and completely reverse type 2 diabetes. Now, it's up to you.

CHAPTER 5 REFERENCES

1. "Leading Causes of Death," U.S. Centers for Disease Control and Prevention final 2009 statistics (http://www.cdc.gov/nchs/fastats/lcod.htm).
2. "Type 1 Diabetes," Children's Hospital of Wisconsin (www.chw.org/display/PPF/DocID/22658/router.asp).
3. Ross Horne, *The Health Revolution* (Avalon Beach, NSW, Australia: Happy Landings, Pty. Ltd., 1980), pp. 311-312.

PART II

The Path to Healing

CHAPTER 6

Restoring the Healing Mechanism

I look forward optimistically to a healthy, happy world as soon as its children are taught the principles of simple and rational living. We must return to nature and nature's God.

—*Luther Burbank (1849–1926)*

> Physicians and the public have exclusively focused on drug
> therapy to the detriment of at least one of the foundations
> of good health—appropriate nutrition.
>
> —*Dr. Mary Keith, St. Michael's Hospital,*
> *Toronto, Ontario*

D r. Max Gerson called the body's defenses its "healing mechanism." He repeatedly observed in his patients that this vital defense had degenerated into a diseased state.

As we have seen, two major problems are present in chronic disease: deficiency and toxicity. If we recognize this fact, we can overcome them both: deficiency through hyperalimentation (the administration of an amount of nutrients that exceeds the appetite) and toxicity through detoxification.

Hyperalimentation

Seriously ill patients are usually unable to eat much. They have a poor appetite, poor digestion and inadequate elimination. **Therefore, Dr. Gerson found that juicing was the answer to providing active nutrients.** Almost every patient is able to drink a freshly prepared glass of juice every hour. In a very few cases, for the first few days on the treatment, the usual hourly 8-ounce glass is reduced to 4 or 6 ounces. Using vitamin and mineral pills doesn't work, since the sick body is unable to assimilate pharmaceutically prepared substances. It accepts only juices and foods freshly prepared from living, raw vegetables and fruit.

Surprisingly, after only a few days of juicing, potassium supplementation and intensive detoxifying, the patients are able to eat three full vegetarian meals prepared from fresh, organic produce. Once the normal intake of 10-13 glasses of juice plus three full meals and fruit snacks is achieved, the patients are actually able to ingest approximately 20 pounds of fresh foods a day. This achieves the needed hyperalimentation.

The juices are freshly prepared, exclusively from organic fruits and vegetables. For the patient suffering from cancer or other serious chronic disease, the juices are as follows:

- 1 glass of orange juice, or grapefruit juice for diabetes patients (at breakfast)

- 5 glasses of a 50/50 mixture of apples and carrots (for patients with high blood sugar, green juices are substituted for 2-3 apple/carrot juices)

- 4 glasses of "green" juices made from lettuce, chard, red cabbage, green pepper and apple

- 3 glasses of straight carrot juice

Of course, there is a reason for the variation in the juices. People assume that citrus is used to supply vitamin C, and indeed the orange or grapefruit juice does contain it; however, other juices are even richer in that important vitamin!

Carrots are extremely rich in numerous minerals and vegetarian protein. The apples in the mixed juice are high in potassium. Apples in the green juices are high in pectin, which makes these juices more easily digestible.

The green juice contains a high level of oxidizing enzymes needed to supply the blood with oxygen—another defense against disease as well as germs and viruses. This juice must be consumed immediately and not be stored since it rapidly loses its enzymes.

The juices are adjusted for some patients (e.g., diabetics, who are given less apple/carrot juice and more green juice until their blood sugar stabilizes). In case of diarrhea, 2 ounces of oatmeal gruel are added to the juices to make them more easily digestible (see Chapter 14, "Understanding Healing Reactions," p. 127).

Meals

For the typical average daily menu of the Gerson patient, see "The Daily Routine," p. 106, in Chapter 11, "Preparing Food and Juices—The Basic

Rules." The particular combination of vegetables used in the "Special Soup or Hippocrates Soup" (see "Special Soup or Hippocrates Soup," p. 108) is specifically used to clear toxins from the kidneys. These vegetables play a major role in detoxifying the body and are helped by the juices and the soup. Other components of the therapy work toward cleansing and detoxifying the liver.

Note that most people are used to the average diet, which invariably contains a lot of sodium. As a result, their taste buds are deadened and, during the first week or so of the treatment, the salt-free Gerson diet tastes "flat" or even "like straw." During that time, patients are urged to use a lot of raw garlic (which should be provided, along with a garlic press) to flavor soup, vegetables, the salad dressing and potatoes. In a few days, the excess sodium is excreted, the taste buds recover and the patients begin to taste and enjoy the food. Actually, the organic produce (correctly prepared instead of boiled in water) is tastier than the commercially grown vegetables. The patients can tell the difference and rarely want to go back to nonorganic foods.

Midday Rest or Sleep

Healing requires energy. Rest is extremely important, so the body can use its still-limited energy for healing. The patient is urged to have at least an hour of total rest after lunch, without watching television or reading; a nap would be most beneficial. A diabetic and/or obese patient should also make room for two to three short walks. He or she should also aim to go to sleep shortly after 10 pm, without watching television or reading. Prayer and/or meditation or some gentle (classical) music can be very soothing and promote peace of mind, sound sleep and healing.

In the early days of the Gerson treatment, the body excretes large amounts of sodium. This can cause the patient to wake up during the night, feeling very thirsty. Since no juice will be available and drinking water is discouraged, the patient should be provided with a thermos of peppermint tea. The argument that tea is essentially water doesn't hold. Peppermint tea helps digestion and promotes the production of stomach acid, while plain water dilutes the already low stomach acid of patients suffering from chronic disease. Besides peppermint tea, chamomile tea is suggested for its calming effect, while valerian tea helps to induce sleep.

Detoxification

It is extremely important to understand that, when the body is being flooded with living nutrients, these readily enter the tissues. At that point, they force the accumulated toxins out of the cells and into the bloodstream. In the course of years of eating the average diet, one cannot help but ingest and accumulate high levels of food additives, residues of pesticides and other toxins that block the liver. Thus, the liver becomes unable to release the extra toxins eliminated from the tissues now being flooded with living nutrients.

The Gerson treatment, using the rapidly detoxifying coffee enemas, clears this problem. It is extremely important to take this detoxification seriously in order to avoid an overload of poisons of the liver. Without the coffee enemas, the additional load of toxins released and flooding the system could poison the liver.

Please note: Do not apply the Gerson Therapy unless coffee enemas are included. (See Chapter 12, "All About Enemas," p. 111.)

Medication

The Gerson Therapy also includes several items of medication (see Table 15-1, "Schedule for Nonmalignant Patients," p. 134, Chapter 15, "The Gerson Therapy for Nonmalignant Diseases"). These are not synthetic drugs aiming to suppress pain or stimulate some organ. They mainly consist of nutrients or substances that the body is not able to produce in its state of deficiency.

Potassium

Dr. Gerson found that the chronically ill patient was severely depleted of potassium. This allowed sodium to invade the cells and cause great damage. While fresh vegetables and especially fruit are high in potassium, it takes a good deal of additional supplementation to restore this essential mineral to the body.

Pancreatin

Pancreatic enzymes are vital for the digestion of foods. They recognize and are able to digest foreign proteins and therefore play an important role in breaking down arterial plaque (atherosclerosis).

Thyroid and Iodine (Lugol's Solution)

These are given to help the thyroid gland produce the thyroid hormone, which controls the metabolism as well as the body's heat production, including fever, and by extension the immune system. The nonsynthetic thyroid supplement, extracted from animal thyroid, and the iodine (Lugol's solution at half strength) are used until the metabolism reaches normal levels.

Niacin (Nicotinic Acid, or Vitamin B₃)

Dr. Gerson states[1] that niacin helps to restore sufficient glycogen to the liver, aids in the protein metabolism and acts to open small arteries and capillaries for improved circulation. While doing this, it often causes the well-known "niacin flush"—the dilation of capillaries that causes redness and mild itching in the area above the chest. This flush can alarm the patient, yet it is totally harmless and usually ceases after the first week or two on the Gerson Therapy. Those who find it annoying are advised to let the tiny (50 mg) niacin tablet melt under their tongue.

Warning: So-called "flush free" or "nonflush" niacin is generally niacinamide and, as such, is useless. Please do not use it. *Niacin does not cause bleeding*; however, if bleeding is present (including during menstruation), it should be discontinued as it could stop the flow from subsiding.

Liver Injection with Vitamin B$_{12}$

Since the healing activity is centered in the liver, and since the liver is toxic and severely damaged, Dr. Gerson used every possible means to help its restoration. The liver extract (3cc) with additional B$_{12}$ (1/10th cc), given daily, supply substances to help restore the liver as well as the bone marrow. The bone marrow produces red blood cells (for oxygen transport throughout the body), white blood cells (which protect the body from foreign invaders) and platelets (needed for forming blood clots to stop bleeding). The injections are given intramuscularly, somewhat behind the hip bone. Dr. Gerson instructed nurses to administer these shots into the "gluteus medius" where it is better absorbed—not the "maximus," which is usually selected, since liver extract is not well assimilated in the fatty tissue of this muscle. Daily shots are given on alternate sides of the body.

Patients are surprised that vitamin C is not supplemented. The reason is that the fresh juices supply this vitamin in very ample amounts, making the pharmaceutical variety unnecessary. Vitamin B$_{12}$ is given to aid in the production of iron-rich red blood cells.

Instructions for Giving Injections[2]

When you return home, you will probably be administering your own injections. During your stay at the Gerson Therapy Center, injections are administered by your medical staff. Learn how to give your own injections by observing, experiencing and asking questions.

1. Assemble items needed:

    - Alcohol

    - Cotton

- Syringe

- Extra needle

- Crude liver extract

- Vitamin B$_{12}$

2.   Bottle: Remove protective metal covers from rubber stopper.

3.   With alcohol swab, clean tops of bottles.

4.   Keep needle and syringe sterile (do not touch).

5.   Turn B$_{12}$ bottle upside down and push syringe needle through stopper. Pull out 0.1 cc (just a few drops) to the first small line on the barrel of syringe. Withdraw needle from B$_{12}$. Draw 3 cc of air into syringe. Turn crude liver bottle upside down and push needle up through center of stopper. Keeping liver extract bottle in an upside-down position, push some air into crude liver bottle and pull some liver extract out, repeating this process until you have pulled out 3 cc of liver extract (pull plunger to first line below 3 cc marking to allow for B$_{12}$).

6.   Remove and discard needle. It is now too dull for injection use.

7.   Screw new needle into syringe. (Use 25-gauge 5/8- or 1-inch needle.) Gently tap the side of syringe to gather bubbles to the top of syringe. When bubbles are gathered, press plunger until a tiny bit of fluid spurts from needle. Syringe is now ready to be used. (Put needle cover on loosely.)

8.   Clean injection area well with alcohol and cotton.

Locating injection area: Locate the ridge of your hipbone (iliac crest) where your side pants seam runs, roughly in the middle of your side. Measure down the width of two fingers and back 1 inch. That is where the needle goes. The needle should go through the fatty tissue into the muscle. Alternate sides with each injection.

Hanson's Modification of Classic Method of Locating Upper Outer Quadrant

9. Spread skin and push needle in.

10. Push plunger down slowly.

11. Pull needle out and rub area with alcohol for 30 seconds. If bleeding occurs, press cotton to wound. It will stop bleeding very shortly.

12. Break needle and disassemble syringe. Keep broken needles in small cardboard box. Tape box shut when full and discard.

13. Clean open liver and B$_{12}$ bottles with alcohol and store in refrigerator. Protect with fresh baggie after each use. Store unopened liver extract bottles in refrigerator.

Exercise

When the Gerson Therapy is dealing with advanced conditions, the patients have to be warned that healing requires energy and therefore rest; however, problems with obesity and diabetes do benefit from exercise.

It is always unwise to overdo, yet with obese patients mild exercise is desirable. Obviously, it will help toward weight loss and improved circulation. In the case of diabetes, it also helps to burn excess sugar and thus activate healing.

If the patient is very ill, weak or has poor muscle control and/or very poor circulation with possible pain in the extremities, it is clear that exercise will have to wait until pain and the lack of control clear up with the organic, salt-free food, juices, enemas and appropriate supplements. The wait is usually not long! The therapy works amazingly fast and severe symptoms generally disappear quickly. Still, one must not force this issue.

Occasionally, patients have arrived at the Gerson hospital with non-healing diabetic lesions (especially around the feet); in rare cases, we see a lack of circulation in toes, which are painful and white instead of pink. These are common symptoms of diabetes. These patients need rest and should not exercise until their situation improves. One woman, who had already been in a wheelchair for about eight years, with serious pain in her legs and unable to stand (let alone walk), was able to get up, stand and even take a few steps in as little as six days! Diabetic lesions are often deep and take longer to "fill in," but the so-called granulation tissue (the cells the body forms when it heals a lesion) becomes clearly visible within a few days.

The "Triad"

In many cases, Dr. Gerson used these three tablets to great effect. Once the patient is sufficiently detoxified, they act more powerfully together than they would separately. The "triad," as we call this combination, continues to be effective for pain relief as well as promoting sound sleep. It consists simply of one regular aspirin, one 500 mg tablet of vitamin C and one 50 mg tablet of the regular niacin, which is part of the patient's normal medication. This combination may be used up to five times a day, every four hours, if needed.

CHAPTER 6 REFERENCES

1. M. Gerson, *A Cancer Therapy: Results of Fifty Cases and The Cure of Advanced Cancer by Diet Therapy: A Summary of Thirty Years of Clinical Experimentation*, 6th ed. (San Diego, CA: Gerson Institute, 1999), p. 209.
2. M. Gerson, *Gerson Therapy Handbook* (San Diego, CA: Gerson Institute, 1999), pp. 12-13.

CHAPTER 7

Why Does the Gerson Therapy Work?

The basic principles of the Gerson protocol are simple and clear, and its practice has been yielding remarkable results for more than 60 years. **However, the question remains: Is there any current scientific research to confirm the methods Dr. Gerson developed partly intuitively, partly through constant study and clinical observation, but without sophisticated research facilities, all those decades ago? Putting it simply, has anyone discovered just why this therapy works?**

The answer is yes. Since Dr. Gerson's death in 1959, a series of eminent scientists and researchers have made discoveries that confirmed one or another of Dr. Gerson's insights and methods. The sum total of these piecemeal discoveries explains why his protocol, used in its entirety, is so effective. We now present a sample of the most striking scientific endorsements.

In the late '70s, the physicist, mathematician and biophysicist Freeman Widener Cope, MD, wrote in a paper stating that, **in cell damage of any kind, the same responses may occur in cells throughout the body: "First the cell will lose potassium, second the cell will accept sodium, and third, the cell will swell with too much water (cellular** edema). **When the cell has swollen with too much water, energy production is inhibited, along with protein synthesis and lipid (fat) metabolism.** *Gerson was able to manipulate tissue damage syndrome, which he recognized clinically in the 1920s, by his dietary management, eliminating sodium, supplementing a high potassium diet with additional potassium amendments and finding a way to remove toxins from the body via the liver.*[1] (Emphasis added.) This is a remarkably concise justification of all of Dr. Gerson's methods, including the strict restriction of protein and fat, which the damaged cell cannot handle, the reason for increased potassium intake and the need for liver detoxification.

Important research justifying Dr. Gerson's withholding of animal protein was carried out by Robert A. Good, MD, of the University of Minnesota, who is known as "the father of modern immunology." He set up a guinea pig experiment, feeding one group of animals protein-free lab chow, while the other group received the normal variety of food. Dr. Good expected to see failure of the animals' immune system on the protein-free regime, but the opposite happened. The guinea pigs' thymus lymphocytes became tremendously active and remained aggressively so for a long time. Dr. Good realized that he had stimulated immunity by the dietary restriction of animal protein, thus confirming the rightness of the Gerson protocol's identical insight.[2]

Gerson patients do receive adequate amounts of easily absorbed plant proteins contained in the fresh vegetable juices, potatoes and oatmeal that are essential parts of their diet. It is a widespread mistake to believe that only animal foods contain protein. On the contrary, food animals, such as cattle, pigs and sheep, are vegetarians!

One of the most important techniques of the Gerson Therapy is detoxification via the liver/bile through the use of coffee enemas. Dr. Gerson knew that these dilate the bile ducts, thus allowing the liver to release toxic accumulations. **His discovery was confirmed more recently by three scientists—Wattenberg, Sparmins and Lam[3]—from the Department of Pathology, University of Minnesota, who showed that rectal coffee administration stimulates an enzyme system (glutathione S-transferase) in the liver, which is able to remove toxic free radicals from the bloodstream. The normal activity of this enzyme is** increased by 600% to 700% by the coffee enema, hence vastly increased detoxification results. Coffee is also rich in potassium, which helps prevent intestinal cramping by boosting the potassium content of deficient smooth muscles in the colon.

CHAPTER 7 REFERENCES

1. Freeman Widener Cope, "Pathology of structured water and associated cations in cells (the tissue damage syndrome) and its medical treatment," *Physiological Chemistry and Physics* 9 (6) (1977): 547-553.
2. Robert A. Good, MD, *The Influence of Nutrition on Development of Cancer Immunity and Resistance to Mesenchymal Diseases* (New York: Raben Press, 1982).
3. V. L. Sparmins, L. K. T. Lam and L. W. Wattenberg, "Proceedings of the American Association of Cancer Researchers and the American Society of Clinical Oncology," *Abstract* 22 (1981): 114, 453.

The Gerson Household

W hether a patient is able to spend some time at a Gerson facility or decides to embark on the therapy at home, the longest part of the healing process—up to two years or more with malignant disease but much less with other chronic conditions—will have to take place in his or her residence. **For the duration of the treatment, the home needs to be turned into a kind of private clinic where everything serves the goal of getting well and nothing is allowed to interfere with that process.**

How do we go about that? Quite simply, we bear in mind that the twin pillars of the Gerson program are nutrition and detoxification. Since the patient is both toxic and nutritionally deficient, as a first task the household has to be cleared of all toxic chemicals and damaging materials or appliances. These are present in vast arrays in most modern households. Chemical cleansers, gadgets and labor-saving devices emitting harmful radiation or so-called electrosmog are used daily and taken for granted. We only get rid of these substances and devices when their dire effects on the body are understood.

The first pillar of the therapy is to provide the patient with hypernutrition and a suitably equipped kitchen. The kitchen is the all-important center where all foods and juices are prepared daily in large amounts.

Let us start by listing the correct equipment for a smoothly running, efficient Gerson kitchen.

Refrigerator

One very large or two average size refrigerators will be needed to store the large quantities of organic produce required. A cool, preferably dark, well-ventilated pantry or laundry room is ideal for storing root vegetables, which don't need refrigeration.

Juice Machines

As freshly made organic juices are one of the most important healing components of the Gerson program, they must be of the best possible quality. It is therefore vital to choose the most efficient juicer—one that will stand up to constant use over two years or so.

There are plenty of models on the market. The simplest and cheapest is the centrifugal type, one of the first to become widely available. It is wasteful, produces deficient, enzyme-poor juice and CANNOT be used for healing.

Another type is the Champion juicer, which extracts more minerals as well as more fluid. However, it is not satisfactory in itself, since what it produces is not so much juice as a mushy layer of vegetables on top of a watery base. **Even so, the Champion juicer can be used, but only as a grinder.** The machine comes with a plate that can be placed under the base where the strainer is usually located, releasing the ground-up pulpy material.

This pulp has to be put through a hand-operated press, based on a hydraulic jack, to squeeze the juice from the pulped vegetables.

The cost of the two items runs at about $600. The Champion juicer is widely available in the United States and in several other countries. For the manual press, contact The Juice Press Factory (www.juicepressfactory.com).

Other machines, imported from Korea and made in the United States, use two interlocking helical blades which grind against each other. They do a better extracting job than the Champion alone and may be used, especially if the patient is not suffering from cancer. However, these "one-process" juicers do not actually conform to Dr. Gerson's instruction to use a two-process method, consisting of a grinder and a press, for obtaining the best juice. These juicers claim to extract more enzymes than the Norwalk (below), but no mention is made of the equally important mineral extraction. The cost of these machines is between $750 and $900.

The best two-process juicer is the Norwalk Hydraulic Press Juicer, which is also most attractively styled with a stainless steel exterior or a wood grain plastic outer cover. Naturally, in either model, all parts of the machine that come in contact with food are made from stainless steel. The Norwalk is fully automatic, with a simple lever activating the press. Well serviced and guaranteed, it is also the most expensive juicer ($2,395 to $2,495). The stainless steel exterior model also has a lever that adjusts it to the 220 to 240 volt current used in Europe. For information, call (800) 405-8423 (outside the United States, call +1 (760) 436-9683) or visit the Norwalk Juicers California Web site (www.nwjcal.com).

For patients on a tight budget, used Norwalk Juicers are sometimes available directly from Norwalk (www.norwalkjuicers.com/used-juicers) or possibly from reseller on eBay (www.eBay.com) or Craigslist (www.craigslist.com).

Taking Care of Your Juice Machine

Aside from your normal routine of maintaining maximum cleanliness in the kitchen, **it is especially important to keep your juicer clean and** free from dried-up juice and/or fibers. Since these are raw, they can easily spoil, dry and attract flies and other insects and germs.

To avoid contamination, the juicer must be cleaned after each use. This should not take up much extra time since those parts of the machine that come in contact with fruits and vegetables are made of stainless steel and are easy to take apart, rinse, dry and reassemble for the next juice.

Use only clean sponges or cloths and reserve them for the juicer alone. **Do not use soap or detergent for each cleansing because it is highly important that not even the smallest amount of soap or cleanser remains on the parts that come in contact with the vegetables.** If you use a Norwalk juicer, remember to wipe the press plate at the top.

The juice cloths should be rinsed carefully in clean—not soapy— water after each pressing and kept in the freezer until the next juicing. It is best to have separate cloths for the apple/carrot or plain carrot juice and for the green juice.

At night, after all the juices have been made, you may use slightly soapy water for the day's final cleansing; afterwards, rinse thoroughly to make sure that no soapy film remains. Even a small residue of soap getting into the juices could cause the patient diarrhea, cramps or worse. The same applies to the juice cloths. Wash them in slightly soapy water and rinse carefully to get rid of any soapy residue. Keep the cloths in the freezer overnight.

If you use a grinder (i.e., a Champion) and a press operated by a hydraulic system, the same rules apply. Keep both machines scrupulously clean and clear of soap.

Stove and Oven: Electric or Gas?

Neither type is ideal. The cooking temperature is easier to control with a gas stove. However, gas burns oxygen, and if the patient spends time in the kitchen, the oxygen-depleted air is likely to prove harmful. The kitchen has to be well ventilated, which may be difficult on cold, winter days. **The installation of a room ozone generator in the kitchen/living area is recommended in order to restore a better oxygen level.**

Caution: If the ozone level is too high, it could be set on fire by open flames.

Electric stoves or ovens are more expensive than gas to operate in most areas of the United States. Their advantage is that they are cleaner and don't use up oxygen. However, the cooking temperature, so very important for the correct preparation of vegetables, is more difficult to control on electric stoves.

Microwave Oven

Because of its speed and apparent efficiency, this gadget has spread to countless kitchens in the United States and elsewhere, without knowing its serious health hazards. Since many microwave ovens carry an "Underwriters Laboratories" guarantee of safety, the general public is led to believe that these ovens are safe to use. This is not the case.

Research carried out in Switzerland[1] and elsewhere has shown that microwaves cause harmful chemical reactions in food, damaging nutrients, producing unnatural molecules and making natural amino acids toxic. The heat is uneven; it doesn't reach the middle of solid food but instead produces "hot spots." Liquids can overheat and cause severe burns when the food is removed. To make things worse, these ovens emit radiation into the kitchen area even when not in use and "cook the cook."[2] **(It is an interesting fact that, for health reasons, microwave ovens were banned in the former Soviet Union as far back as 1976!)**[3] If you own one, get rid of it. If it is not removable, unplug it and don't be tempted to use it under any circumstances.

Pots and Utensils

Any contact of food with aluminum causes small amounts (or with some vegetables, such as tomatoes, large amounts) of aluminum to be dissolved and released into the food. This metal is highly toxic;

it causes brain damage and is believed to play a role in causing Alzheimer's.[4]

Discard any and all aluminum items and don't allow aluminum foil to come into contact with food. Use stainless steel pots, preferably with heavy "waterless" bottoms, or glass (Pyrex®) or enameled cast iron pots. Stainless steel cooking utensils or wooden spoons are best. Use silver flatware, if available (small amounts of colloidal silver, released from silver forks, spoons and knives are valuable stimulants for the immune system).

Do not use pressure cookers; they work at a very high temperature, which damages nutrients. One of the basic Gerson rules is to cook food very slowly, at a low temperature, to avoid such damage. The glaze used on some crockpots is toxic[5]—best to steer clear of them.

Distillers

Surprising though this may sound, Gerson patients don't drink water. There are two reasons for this. On the one hand, their daily intake of many glasses of freshly made organic juices and fluid-rich soup, salads and fruit provide them with all the top-quality nutritious liquid they need. **On the other hand, water would only dilute their already deficient digestive juices without supplying any nutrients.** However, water is used in the Gerson Therapy in cooking—to make soups, teas and, of course, enemas—and it is vitally important to ensure the purity of this water.

There are various filter systems on the market, including reverse osmosis, which can only be used if the local water supply is guaranteed free from highly harmful fluoride. **The safest way to ensure freedom from impurities, toxic chemicals and, above all, fluoride is to set up a home distiller.**

Many kinds of distillers are available in various price ranges. Choice must depend on cost and on the amount of water the household may need. The patient alone will use 2 to 3 gallons in every 24-hour period, and more if other family members also eat Gerson food and/or wish to use enemas.

A distiller needs an electric connection and an extra water faucet, and many patients install theirs in the laundry room or garage. **The machine needs to be detached and cleaned every three days.** Seeing the sludge left behind will convince anyone of the need to purify water as thoroughly as possible.

Distillation works by heating water to the point of becoming steam, which is run through a tube that causes it to cool and condense back into water. Since minerals, various impurities and additives do not turn into steam, they stay behind, leaving the cooled, condensed steam free from harmful components. However, volatile liquids, such as benzene fractions, also boil away and are condensed back into the purified water.

To remove such items, make sure the distiller you choose contains a carbon filtration system, so that when the condensed water drips back into a fresh container, it passes through the carbon filter, which removes the unwanted volatile items.

It is sometimes claimed by health professionals that distilled water "removes minerals from the body" and shouldn't be used,[6] but they are wrong. The minerals found in water (e.g., sodium or calcium) are generally inorganic and are therefore poorly absorbed or downright harmful. On the other hand, the patient is virtually flooded with the easily absorbed organic minerals contained in the large amount of juices drunk throughout the day; the "loss" of minerals contained in tap water is actually a gain.

Cleaning Chemicals

Cleanliness is of course all important in the Gerson household but, as stated before, **special care must be taken not to use toxic products. Here are the ones to avoid:**

Chlorine

Chlorine is not only bleach but also a powerful disinfectant, able to kill or control all kinds of germs. For that reason, it is present in almost all kitchen cleansers (and in swimming pools and tap water!). **Chlorine is**

harsh and unsafe, able to displace iodine from the thyroid gland and must be avoided. There are a few kitchen cleansers that do not contain chlorine, so try to find one. You can also produce your own by mixing half malt vinegar with half water and decanting it into a spray-pump bottle to clean glass or polish kitchen surfaces, but keep it off wood. Plain soap and hot water are also recommended.

To remove lime scale, soak a piece of cotton in white vinegar, wrap it around the faucets in your kitchen or bathroom and leave it for 30 minutes. Wash it off with soap and water.

Clean stainless steel pans with olive oil. The result is stunning, but use the oil sparingly and be careful to clean it all off.

Solvents

Paint solvents, grease or glue solvents are all toxic and damaging to the patient. If one has to be used, take it outside and don't allow it to evaporate in the kitchen.

Dishwasher Soap

Most dishwashers are equipped with two wash cycles followed by one rinse cycle. Since the Gerson Therapy does not involve the use of greasy food or baking dishes, **it is best to use one wash cycle and ensure that the soap is cleared by using two rinse cycles.** In that way, the dishwasher soap should be completely eliminated, with no toxic residue remaining on dishes.

Laundry Soap and Bleach

If the laundry is washed in a washing machine, the same applies to dishwasher soap. You can use any appropriate soap and even add bleach, if needed, as long as it is inside the machine and the patient doesn't smell it. **(If the patient can smell it, he or she is getting some into their system.)** Make very sure that the laundry is thoroughly rinsed, possibly running a second rinse cycle.

Fabric Softeners

These should be avoided, whether in liquid form or as drying sheets. Either way, they leave a chemical film, which never washes out completely. They are also irritating to sensitive individuals (e.g., asthma sufferers). As a harmless alternative, add 1/4 cup of distilled white vinegar to the wash cycle. This softens your clothes and also gets rid of static cling. If you are washing delicate items (e.g., those marked "hand wash"), use a mild soap and wear rubber gloves.

Dry Cleaning

As this is done outside the home, it doesn't directly affect the patient. However, when dry-cleaned items are brought home, it is wise to leave them outdoors without their plastic covers to let them air out and get rid of any remaining chemicals.

Aerosols and Sprays

Do not use any of these. Once the spray is distributed in the air, it is impossible to avoid inhaling it. Obviously, the toxic pesticide sprays are the most dangerous. However, any cleaning chemicals (e.g., window cleaners and oven cleaners) that are sprayed will go into the air and be inhaled.

If a window cleaner is used, pour a little on a cloth and wipe the window clean without spraying. As a suggestion, windows can be cleaned and completely streak free by pouring white vinegar on some slightly crumpled newspaper and wiping the window (with light pressure) until clean.

Oven cleaning is not much of a problem, since the Gerson food is clear of fats and doesn't cause deposits on the oven walls.

The Bathroom

Chlorine-containing cleansers should not be used in the bathroom. Disinfect with 3% commercial hydrogen peroxide.

It is important to note that your skin is a semipermeable membrane, which means that everything you put on your skin is absorbed into your body. This includes all of the chemicals contained in your soaps, shampoos, toothpaste, creams, balms, cosmetics, fragrances, aftershaves, colognes, convenience wipes and more. **As much as possible, patients on the Gerson Therapy should only use organic soaps and shampoos with a minimum amount of chemicals and fragrances.** Gerson patients should make sure to avoid all spray deodorizers, antiperspirants and underarm deodorants.

Men should use old-style spreadable shaving soaps, not products that come in aerosol cans or sprays. Avoid aerosol aftershaves and perfumes and any scented lotions. Only use plain, white, unscented toilet paper.

There are numerous organic soaps and shampoos available today, and your local organic food store should have a full range for you to pick from. Also, a quick search on the Internet will provide an abundance of chemical-free items that will suit your personal preferences.

Dental Care

Brushing and Flossing

Good dental hygiene is important on the Gerson Therapy. **Patients should take care to brush and floss regularly** as bacteria may form in between teeth and gums and may enter the bloodstream. Patients are also advised to rinse with distilled water and dry brush after each juice to prevent cavities that may arise from natural sugar in the carrots and apples that accumulates on the teeth and around the gums.

Fluoride Toothpaste

Patients must not use fluoride toothpaste. The fluoride in toothpaste is as toxic as the fluoride in water, and will be absorbed by the mucous membranes in the mouth. To illustrate this point, the packaging of toothpaste containing fluoride displays a warning that if you eat or swallow more than a pea-sized dollop of toothpaste, you should call your local poison control center immediately.

> # WARNING
> **Keep out of the reach of Children under 6 years of age.**
> **If you accidentaly swallow more than is used for**
> **brushing, get medical help or contact a poison**
> **control center right away.**
> **When using this product, if irritation occurs**
> **discontinue use.**

Mercury Amalgam Fillings

Warning regarding the removal of mercury amalgam fillings: Gerson patients must not have their silver amalgam fillings removed until they have been on the therapy at least nine to 12 months. Even with the best precautions, the high-speed drills used during the removal process will:

- Release poisonous mercury gas that will be inhaled by the patient

- Create microparticles of mercury amalgam that may be absorbed in the mouth, inhaled and/or swallowed

- Create medium-sized particles of mercury amalgam that can be swallowed

Mercury is a poisonous neurotoxin, and even small amounts ingested during the removal of fillings can make normal healthy individuals very sick. With Gerson patients, it can have serious consequences.

Polishing Fillings During Dental Cleanings

Patients should never allow their "silver" amalgam fillings to be polished, cleaned or abraded for any reason. This will remove the body's natural covering material and the slight surface oxidation that helps to keep some the mercury from leaching into the body.

Baking Soda

A question we receive quite often is whether patients can use baking soda in place of toothpaste. The answer is NO! What is baking soda? Sodium bicarbonate—a sodium-based compound—must be avoided as it will be absorbed in the mouth, sabotaging the healing process.

Living Area

Many kinds of toxic damage can be caused inadvertently in the living room. **One possible culprit is furniture polish, which contains solvent and must be banished.** Carpet cleaning presents another potential hazard. Do not use (or allow cleaning services to use) chemical cleaners, only soapy solutions.

Very serious toxic damage has been caused by new carpeting,[7] most of which is impregnated with toxic pesticides or other chemicals to resist staining. If it is absolutely necessary to install new carpeting, track down nontoxic kinds. Several manufacturers have been sued[8] for their carpets causing allergic reactions in sensitive people and, as a result, nontoxic carpets are now being produced.

An even more dangerous process is termite extermination. Some exterminators use a whole house cover and spread gas throughout the building. When the covers are removed, fresh air is allowed back in, but a lot of poison is left behind in upholstered furniture, carpets and drapes. It takes some six months or so to outgas! There are other nontoxic methods available (e.g., find out about the freezing approach).

Living room areas are often routinely treated to "air fresheners" via sprays or a chemical solid. Do not use either.

Whole House Painting

No part of the inside of the house should be painted while the patient is recovering. Walls may be washed down with mild soap; stains can be removed with a nontoxic cleanser. The house may not look perfect but, for the time being, the patient's recovery must be given absolute priority.

Outdoor Garden Sprays/Agricultural Pesticides

Some areas of daily life are beyond the caregiver's control, such as neighbors who spray their gardens with pesticides. If and when this happens, make sure that all windows are closed, and use the room air cleaner and ozone generator to protect the patient. A similar problem is caused by pesticide spraying of agricultural areas in the vicinity. In one such case, the recovering patient had a serious reaction and suffered a recurrence until she moved away (to live with her sister) for the time being, where she recovered again.

CHAPTER 8 REFERENCES

1. Hans Hertel and Bernard H. Blanc, "Microwave Ovens" (Vol. 22, No. 2) and "Microwaves the Best Article Yet," Price-Pottenger Nutrition Foundation, *PPNF Journal* 24 (2) (Summer 2000).
2. Ibid.
3. Ibid.
4. Virginie Rondeau, Daniel Commenges, Hélène Jacqmin-Gadda and Jean-François Dartigues, "Relation between Aluminum Concentrations in Drinking Water and Alzheimer's Disease: An 8-year Follow-up Study," *American Journal of Epidemiology* 152 (2000): 59-66.
5. Dixie Farley, "Dangers of Lead Still Linger," U.S. Food and Drug Administration, *FDA Consumer* (January-February 1998) (www.cfsan.fda.gov/~dms/fdalead.html).
6. P. Airola, *How To Get Well* (Phoenix: Health Plus Publishers, 1974).
7. Cindy Duehring, "Carpet Concerns, Part Four: Physicians Speak Up As Medical Evidence Mounts," Environmental Access Research Network (Minot, ND) (www.holisticmed.com/carpet/tc4.txt).

8. Fluoride Action Network, Pesticide Project, Class Action Suit-PFOA (www.fluoridealert.org/pesticides/effect.pfos.classaction.htm).

CHAPTER 9

Forbidden Foods

A McDonald's "Breakfast for Under a Dollar"
actually costs much more than that. You have to
factor in the cost of coronary bypass surgery.

—George Carlin

Just as some foods, brilliantly combined in the Gerson protocol, are great healers, others are strictly excluded from the patient's diet. In his classic book, *A Cancer Therapy—Results of Fifty Cases,*[1] Dr. Gerson gives a long list of "Forbidden Foods." Actually, "Forbidden Items" would be a more accurate title, since the list is not limited to foodstuffs only. Newcomers to the Gerson program are understandably puzzled by some of these prohibitions, banning foods that are routinely eaten and even considered wholesome by the average "normal" citizen, so let's see why they must be excluded. Rules and regulations are easier to follow if we know the reasons behind them.

In fact, today's list of banned substances is longer than Dr. Gerson's original one. Since he wrote his book half a century ago, many changes have occurred that make healthy living increasingly difficult. The huge development of the food industry—with its vast range of additives, freely used in the ever-wider assortment of convenience foods—has changed people's eating habits for the worse, exposing consumers to the ill effects of what are politely called food cosmetics.

One of the worst—the highly toxic[2] sugar substitute aspartame, sold as NutraSweet®, Spoonful®, Equal®—is contained in some 6,000[3] processed foods found on grocery shelves. Last, but far from least, all processed foods contain salt, the very substance that causes tissue damage syndrome and stimulates tumor growth.[4]

Added to this, the products of industrial agriculture carry heavy residues of toxic pesticides, herbicides, fungicides, growth promoters, hormones, antibiotics and any one of the thousands of substances allowed to be used by the FDA,[5] which are supposed to be harmless. **Indeed, some of these substances tested singly may prove to be harmless but, in combination with others, which is how people consume them in the real world, they add up to a poisonous cocktail.** Let's remember that all these chemicals are toxic and damaging to the liver, the very organ which the Gerson Therapy endeavors to heal and restore.

These are the two basic rules for Gerson patients:

- All processed foods, whether they are canned, jarred, bottled, frozen, salted, refined, sulphured, smoked, pickled, irradiated, microwaved or otherwise treated, must be strictly avoided.

- Only fruits and vegetables certified as organic must be used, for they are free of agricultural poisons and are grown in healthy soil, which contains all the necessary vitamins, enzymes, minerals, trace elements and microorganisms that are needed for optimum health.

Admittedly, these days even organically cultivated soil does not contain the same level of useful minerals as it did even 15 years ago, but the great amount of organic food and juices that a Gerson patient is given daily makes up for the deficiencies.

As for the forbidden items, the harmful effects of tobacco and alcohol are too well known to need explanation. Next, sodium (salt) and fats of all kinds, except flaxseed oil, must be avoided. This, of course, brings into the group of forbidden foods many items that contain one or both of these two banned substances (e.g., avocados are rich in natural oil, which is fat). If you bear in mind the ban on fats and salt, the following list will make sense without detailed explanations.

To simplify matters even further, let's repeat loud and clear: Only foods that contribute to health and healing are allowed; all else is banned.

Forbidden Foods and Nonfood Items

- All processed foods (premade, heat and eat, ready to eat and prepackaged industrial foods)
- Alcohol
- Avocados
- Berries (except currants)
- Bicarbonate of soda (baking soda) in foods, toothpaste and gargle
- Bottled and canned commercial beverages (soft drinks)
- Cake, candy, chocolate and all kinds of sweets (high sugar and fats; no nutritional value)
- Cheese
- Cocoa
- Coffee for drinking
- Cosmetics, hair dyes and permanents
- Cream
- Cucumber (poorly digested)
- Dried fruit (if sulphured or glazed with oil)
- Drinking water (see the section on distillers in Chapter 8, "The Gerson Household," p. 84)

- Epsom salts (also for foot baths)
- Fats and oils (sole exception: flaxseed oil, as prescribed)
- Flour (white and wholemeal; also flour products such as pasta)
- Fluoride, in water and toothpaste
- Herbs (except permitted ones) (see Chapter 11, "Preparing Food and Juices—The Basic Rules," p. 103)
- Ice cream and sherbet (artificial flavors, sweeteners and cream)
- Legumes (only occasional use in latter part of therapy)
- Milk (also defatted or low fat)
- Mushrooms (fungi, not vegetables)
- Nuts (high in fats; wrong configuration of proteins)
- Orange and lemon rind (contains aromatic oils)
- Pickles
- Pineapples (high in aromatics)
- Salt and all salt substitutes
- Soy and all soy products (e.g., tofu, soy milk and flour)
- Most spices (high in aromatics)
- Sugar (refined white)
- Tea (black and green if caffeinated; black tea is high in natural fluoride)

Dr. Gerson's total ban on soy and all soy products may sound surprising at first, since soy has the much-publicized reputation of being an ideal vegetarian food (i.e., high in protein and low in fat and cholesterol). It is also consumed in the Far East where cancer incidence is considerably lower than in the West.

However, the truth behind this commercially motivated publicity is very different (soy is very big business in the United States, where 60% of supermarket foods contain some form of it). In fact, soy is high in oil and contains at least 30 allergy-causing proteins, which can cause severe damage[6] to susceptible individuals. Soy also contains phytic acid, which blocks the uptake of important minerals; enzyme inhibitors, which annul the healing power of the vital oxidizing enzymes contained in the juices; and a clot-promoting substance, which causes red blood cells to clump together—ample justification for the total exclusion of soy from the Gerson protocol.

Please note: **Two "home-grown" foods—sprouted seeds and wheatgrass juice—which became fashionable some 20 years ago and are considered wholesome and nutritious, must not be used by Gerson patients.** Our experience has shown that, unfortunately, both have harmful side effects.

Sprouts were eaten in large amounts by two Gerson patients at our hospital instead of the usual salads at lunch and dinner. Within a short time, both developed recurrences of their primary diseases (i.e., lupus and cervical cancer) after being symptom-free for months. Other lupus patients, getting sprouts from the hospital kitchen in their salads and juices, stopped responding to the treatment and even got worse.

Shortly afterwards, researchers[7] discovered that sprouts contain immature proteins, called L-canavanine, which suppress the immune system. At the Gerson hospital, sprouts were immediately banned and the earlier problems disappeared at once. All past patients were also advised to stop using sprouts in their diet.

Wheatgrass juice contains many valuable nutrients, but it is difficult to digest, tends to irritate the stomach and can only be taken in 1-ounce portions. Used as a rectal implant, it can cause serious irritation. Besides, the Gerson green juice (consisting of salad greens, chard, a little green pepper, some red cabbage and an apple per 8-ounce glass) (see Chapter 11, "Preparing Food and Juices—The Basic Rules," p. 103) is highly digestible, contains similar nutrients and can be enjoyed in four 8-ounce portions a day without unpleasant side effects—excellent reasons for not using wheatgrass juice.

Temporarily Forbidden Foods While on Gerson Healing Program

- Butter
- Cottage cheese (salt-free, defatted)
- Eggs
- Fish
- Meat
- Yogurt (and other fermented milk products)

Forbidden Personal and Household Items

- Aerosols of all types
- Carpeting (new)
- Chemical cleansers (see Chapter 8, "The Gerson Household," p. 79)
- Chlorine bleach
- Cosmetics
- Ointments
- Paint (fresh)
- Perfumes
- Pesticide sprays
- Wood preservatives

CHAPTER 9 REFERENCES

1. M. Gerson, *A Cancer Therapy: Results of Fifty Cases and The Cure of Advanced Cancer by Diet Therapy: A Summary of Thirty Years of Clinical Experimentation,* 6th ed. (San Diego, CA: Gerson Institute, 1999).

2. Aspartame (NutraSweet®) Toxicity Info Center (www.holisticmed.com/aspartame); *see also* H. J. Roberts, MD, "Does Aspartame Cause Human Brain Cancer?," *Journal of Advancement in Medicine* 4 (4) (Winter 1991).

3. Joseph Mercola, MD, "Can Rumsfeld 'Defend' Himself Against Aspartame Lawsuit?" (www.mercola.com/2005/jan/12/rumsfeld_aspartame.htm); *see also* Note 2 (Roberts), supra.

4. Freeman Widener Cope, "A medical application of the Ling Association-Induction Hypothesis: the high potassium, low sodium diet of the Gerson cancer therapy," *Physiological Chemistry and Physics* 10 (5) (1978): 465-468.

5. Healthy Eating Adviser: Food Additives (www.healthyeatingadvisor.com/food-additives.html) (updated 2006).

6. "Soy Dangers Summarised," SoyOnlineService (www.soyonlineservice.co.nz/03summary.htm).

7. M. R. Malinow, E. J. Bardana, Jr., B. Pirofsky, S. Craig and P. McLaughlin, "Systemic lupus erythematosus-like syndrome in monkeys fed alfalfa sprouts: role of a nonprotein amino acid," *Science* 216 (4544) (Apr. 23, 1982): 415-417.

CHAPTER 10

Happy Foods

Even the highest medicine can cure only eight
or nine out of 10 sicknesses. The sicknesses that
medicine cannot cure can be cured only by foods.

—The Yellow Emperor's Classic of Internal
Medicine *(Chinese, circa 400 B.C.)*

Food is Better Medicine than Drugs

*—Title of book by leading British
nutritionist Patrick Holford*

"So what *is* there to eat?" asks the startled newcomer to the Gerson way of life, after reading the list of forbidden foods in the preceding chapter. That is an important question to ponder. It shows how alienated one can become from a natural way of eating and, above all, from the huge range of available plant foods, rightly called the vegetable kingdom (which, in this instance, also includes fruits). It is a fair guess that the majority of people in the so-called developed world regard vegetables as no more than incidentals that accompany a main course of fish or meat, while fruits are only considered if there is no dessert offered. This is the moment to think again—and to make some delightful discoveries.

The fact is that plant foods, which are the basis of the Gerson regime, are superior to animal-based ones. Besides being lighter, more pure and easier to digest and absorb, each one contains a subtle mixture of vitamins, enzymes, minerals and trace elements, which work in synergy (i.e., in cooperation) and supply the depleted organism with valuable nutrients. Only when the nonhealing—in fact, harmful—food items are excluded, the wide range and variety of plant foods become clear. It is their usefulness as well as their beauty that need to be acknowledged.

Try to look at a display of fresh, organic fruits and vegetables with the eyes of an artist. Note the glowing colors and varied shapes of golden carrots, deep red cabbages, creamy cauliflowers with their light green collars, beige pears, multicolored apples and translucent green grapes— the range is vast, and eye appeal adds a great deal to the enjoyment of the produce.

There is another happy surprise that awaits the novice explorer of the vegetable kingdom: the discovery of the true flavor of vegetables and fruits. At first, without salt and pepper, plant foods taste bland—and, frankly, boring—but they are neither. However, a lifetime of excessive use of salt deadens the taste buds of the tongue until they are unable to convey the true taste of any food, and even the salt intake has to be continually increased to have any effect. On the salt-free Gerson regime, it takes a week or so for the paralyzed taste buds to recover. Once that happens, fruits and vegetables suddenly begin to taste more interesting. At the same time, one's sense of smell also becomes more acute and contributes to the enjoyment of every meal.

"Let your food be your medicine, and let your medicine be your food," said Hippocrates, the father of modern medicine, some 2,500 years ago. [Emphasis added.] We might add, "Let your medicine consist of happy foods only!"

CHAPTER 11

Preparing Food and Juices —The Basic Rules

A first-rate soup is more
creative than a second-rate painting.

—Abraham Maslow

Assuming that your kitchen is now fully equipped for your healing Gerson routine, and that you have banished from your home all forbidden foods and substances, the moment has come to find out about the all-important task of food preparation. The rules are simple, but they must be observed faithfully to secure the best results.

All food must be organic and as fresh as possible. Ideally, we should be able to gather fresh, living food from our own organic gardens; unfortunately, this is not an ideal world and we must compromise. The next best thing is to shop frequently for salad and leaf vegetables in smallish amounts so there is no need to keep them for any length of time. Apples, pears, oranges and root vegetables can be stored for a while without significant loss of quality.

The two most important basic rules of food preparation are the following:

- All foods must be prepared with great care in order to preserve nutrients as much as possible. **Cooking must be slow, using low heat**; *high temperatures alter nutrients in vegetables and cause them to be less easily absorbed.* Vegetables should not be peeled—valuable nutrients are contained in or immediately underneath their skins—and only washed or well scrubbed. Except for potatoes, corn and whole beets, which have to be boiled in sufficient water, vegetables are cooked with the minimum of water or soup stock (see "Special Soup or Hippocrates Soup," p. 108) or on a bed of sliced onions and tomatoes, which release enough moisture to keep the vegetables from burning. **Remember that oxidation, with loss of nutrients, sets in as soon as you cut into a vegetable or fruit; only start chopping when you are ready to cook.**

- Food must be tasty, varied and enjoyable to make up for being very different from the so-called normal Western diet. Variety helps to stimulate appetite. It also supplies a wide range of minerals and trace elements needed by the body to heal. Remember the importance of eye appeal! Salads in particular can be made truly tempting by mixing green leaves with chopped tomatoes and multicolored peppers, adding radishes and a smattering of chives. (For further ideas, see Chapter 22, "Recipes," p. 165.)

A small vase of flowers on the dining table can work wonders in making the meal taste even better.

The Gerson diet strikes a fine balance between raw and cooked foods. The ample main meals may suggest to some patients that much of their food is cooked, but this is not the case. Meals begin with huge helpings of raw salad and end with raw fruit, and the daily ration of 13 glasses of freshly made juice is as raw as can be. **Cooked foods are necessary. Dr. Gerson's experience showed that patients do not digest well if given only raw foods along with the juices.** In fact, cooked foods provide additional variety and enable patients to eat more than they would on an exclusively raw diet. They also supply soft bulk, which promotes the digestion of the raw foods and juices.

The most popular item on the list of cooked foods is the "Special Soup or Hippocrates Soup" (p. 108) that helps to detoxify the kidneys and is highly comforting, especially in cold weather. All cooked foods serve as a kind of "blotting paper" in the stomach, helping to deal with the constant intake of large amounts of juice. Even so, cooked foods only account for some 3 to 4 pounds of the patient's daily consumption, while raw foods, mostly made into juices, represent some 17 pounds!

The All-Important Juices

Only four kinds of juice are used in the treatment of all categories of patients, except for a few minor exceptions. The basic juices are:

- **Apple/carrot juice**
- **Carrot-only juice**
- **Green juice**
- **Orange juice**

Occasionally, for special cases, a different juice may have to be substituted. For example, diabetics receive grapefruit juice instead of orange juice, since grapefruit contains less sugar; sometimes a fruit juice, such as apple juice, is given to patients with collagen diseases who should not drink citrus juice.

Apple/Carrot Juice

Use approximately 8 ounces each of carrots and apples. Wash and brush (do not peel), grind to a pulp and place in a cloth supplied with the press-type juicer to press. Serve and drink immediately.

Carrot-Only Juice

Use approximately 10-12 ounces of carrots. Wash and brush (do not peel), grind to a pulp and place in a cloth supplied with the press-type juicer to press. Serve and drink immediately.

Green Juice

Use romaine, red leaf lettuce, endive, escarole, two to three leaves of red cabbage, young inner beet tops, Swiss chard, a quarter of a small green pepper and watercress. Add one medium apple when grinding. Procure as many of these materials as possible. If some of the above items are not available, do not use substitutes, such as spinach or celery. Grind the material to a pulp and place in a cloth for pressing. This juice must be drunk immediately since its enzymes die quickly.

Orange (or Grapefruit) Juice

Use only a reamer-type juicer, electric or hand operated. **Do not squeeze the peel of the fruit. The aromatic oils contained in the skin are harmful and would interfere with the treatment.**

The Daily Routine

The typical average daily menu of the Gerson patient is as follows:

Breakfast

- A large bowl of oatmeal cooked in distilled water and sweetened with a little honey or dried fruit, presoaked (soak overnight in cold water, or pour boiling water over them)

- An 8-ounce glass of freshly squeezed orange juice

- Some additional raw or stewed fruit

- *Optional:* a slice of toasted, unsalted, organic rye bread

Lunch

- A large plate of mixed raw salad with flaxseed oil dressing (see the Flaxseed Oil and Lemon Juice Dressing recipe in Chapter 22, "Recipes," p. 175)
- 8 to 10 ounces of the "Special Soup or Hippocrates Soup" (see p. 108)
- Baked, boiled, mashed or otherwise prepared potato
- 1 to 2 freshly cooked vegetables
- Raw or stewed fruit for dessert

Dinner

- Follows the same order as lunch, but is varied with different vegetables and fruit for dessert

Please note: Either at lunch or dinner, and after the patient has consumed the necessary foods, *he or she may eat a second slice of unsalted, organic rye bread. However, bread should not satisfy the appetite or take the place of essential foods.*

Basic Recipes to Start You Off

For a full range of Gerson recipes, please see Chapter 22, "Recipes," p. 165. The following instructions are only meant to introduce the most fundamental items of the patient's essential daily menu.

Breakfast

For one person, put 5 ounces of rolled oats into 12 ounces of **distilled water**. Start with cold water, bring to a boil and let simmer for 6 to 8 minutes, stirring occasionally. Meanwhile, squeeze orange juice and add any prescribed medication(s) (see Chapter 13, "Medications," p. 121). Serve the oatmeal with presoaked (soak overnight in cold water, or pour boiling water over them and leave for a couple of hours until plump), unsulphured dried fruit (e.g., apricots, apple rings, prunes, raisins and mango), or use raw or stewed apple or stewed plums, or fresh fruit in season (e.g., peaches, nectarines, grapes or pears) **Do not use berries.** Up to 2 teaspoons a day of permitted sweeteners (e.g., honey, maple syrup, spray-dried cane juices sold as sucanat (an organic dried cane sugar) and rapadura, or unsulphured molasses) may be used.

Lunch

For the salad, cut up, slice and mix varied lettuces, such as red leaf lettuce, Romaine, escarole, salad bowl and endive. Add to the mixture chopped green onions, radishes, a little celery, some tomatoes, cauliflower florets, slices of green pepper and watercress. For the dressing (see the Flaxseed Oil and Lemon Juice Dressing recipe in Chapter 22, "Recipes," p. 175), mix 1 tablespoon of flaxseed oil (during the first month of the therapy; afterwards, reduce to 2 teaspoons) with apple cider or red wine vinegar, or lemon or lime juice. Add garlic to taste.

"Special Soup or Hippocrates Soup" (below) is to be eaten twice daily throughout the treatment. To save time and effort, prepare enough for two days (i.e., four portions). It will keep in the refrigerator overnight for the next day.

Special Soup or Hippocrates Soup

1 medium celery root, if available
    (if not, 3 to 4 celery branches (i.e., pascal))
1 medium parsley root (rarely available; may be omitted)
2 small or one large leek (if not available, use 2 small onions instead)
2 medium onions
garlic to taste
    (may also be squeezed raw into the hot soup instead of cooking it)
small amount of parsley
1-1/2 pounds tomatoes (or more, if desired)
1 pound potatoes

Wash and scrub vegetables and cut into slices or 1/2-inch cubes. Put in large pot, add water to just cover vegetables, bring to a boil, then cook slowly on low heat for 1-1/2 to 2 hours until all the vegetables are soft. Pass through a food mill to remove fibers. Let soup cool before storing in refrigerator.

Please note: **Many spices are high in aromatic acids, which are irritants and are likely to counteract the healing reaction.** This is why only the following mild spices are permitted, to be used in *very small doses*: **allspice, anise, bay leaves, coriander, dill, fennel, mace, marjoram, rosemary, saffron, sage, sorrel, summer savory, tarragon and thyme. In addition, chives, garlic, onion and parsley may be used in larger amounts. Two herb teas—chamomile and peppermint—are frequently used by Gerson patients.** For details, please see Chapter 12, "All About Enemas," p. 111, and Chapter 14, "Understanding Healing Reactions," p. 127.

All About Enemas

To the uninitiated, the coffee enema is the most surprising and apparently bizarre element of the Gerson Therapy. Critics like to attack and ridicule it without bothering to find out its purpose and function. Yet, without this simple tool of detoxification, the Gerson method wouldn't work. Before going into details, let us make clear why this is so.

The moment a patient is put on the full therapy, the combined effect of the food, the juices and the medication causes the immune system to flush out accumulated toxins from the body tissues. This great clearing-out procedure carries the risk of over-burdening and poisoning the liver—the all-important organ of detoxification, which is bound to be already damaged and debilitated.

Generally speaking, any kind of enema introduces a substance into the rectum in order to empty the bowel or to administer nutrients or drugs. **It is a medical procedure of great antiquity.** Hippocrates, the

Greek "father of modern medicine," prescribed water enemas for several conditions some 2,600 years ago. In India, enemas were recommended for inner cleansing by Patanjali, author of the first written work on yoga, in around 200 B.C. According to tradition, the ibis (a sacred bird of ancient Egypt associated with wisdom) used to administer itself an enema with its long curved beak.

Closer to our own time, a lady in the court of King Louis XIV of France is reported to have taken an enema under her voluminous skirts, and "Le Malade Imaginaire" (i.e., "The Hypochondriac," in Moliere's play of the same title) enjoyed an enema on stage. It is only in recent times, and mainly in English-speaking countries, that this simple and safe cleansing method had fallen into disuse.

The use of coffee as enema material began in Germany towards the end of World War I (1914–1918). The country was blockaded by the Allies and many essential goods—among them, morphine—were not available, yet trainloads of wounded soldiers kept arriving at field hospitals, needing surgery. The surgeons had barely enough morphine to dull the pain of the operations but none to help patients endure the postsurgical pain; all they could do was to use water enemas.

Although, owing to the blockade, coffee was in short supply, there was plenty of it around to help the surgeons stay awake during their long spells of duty. The nurses, desperate to ease their patients' pain, began to pour some of the leftover coffee into the enema buckets. They figured that, since it helped the surgeons (who drank it), the soldiers (who didn't) would also benefit from it. Indeed, the soldiers reported pain relief.

This accidental discovery came to the attention of two medical researchers—Professors Meyer and Huebner at the University of Goettingen[1] in Germany—who went on to test the effects of rectally infused caffeine on rats. **They found that the caffeine, traveling via the hemorrhoidal vein and the portal system to the liver, opened up the bile ducts, allowing the liver to release accumulated toxins.** This observation was confirmed 70 years later, in 1990, by Peter Lechner, MD,[2] oncologist surgeon at the District Hospital of Graz, Austria, after running a six-year controlled test on cancer patients following a slightly modified version of the Gerson Therapy. **In his report, he quotes independent laboratory results, identifying the two components of coffee that play the major role in detoxifying the liver.** (See Chapter 7, "Why Does the Gerson Therapy Work?," p. 75.)

Dr. Gerson became aware of the benefits of enemas early in developing his treatment, and they have remained a cornerstone of his therapy to this day. It is important to realize that, while the patient is holding the coffee enema in his or her colon for the suggested 12 to 15 minutes, the body's entire blood supply passes through the liver every three minutes (i.e., four to five times in all), carrying poisons picked up from the tissues. These are then released through the bile ducts due to the stimulation of the caffeine.

However, in order to leave the body, these toxins still have to travel through the small intestine (25 to 27 feet), through the colon (4 to 5 feet) and out via the rectum and the anus. Naturally, on this long trip, a small amount of the released toxins is reabsorbed into the system and can cause the patient discomfort, especially in the early phase of the therapy, when detoxification had only just started. This is the reason why, in the beginning, five or more enemas are taken daily.

Important warning: **Although high colonics have become fashionable among some celebrities, they must not be used by Gerson patients.** Dr. Gerson had stated this very clearly, and we can only reiterate his conclusion. In high colonics, up to 5 quarts of water are forced into the whole length of the large intestine, under pressure that can easily distend it. When the water is released, it washes out the fluids, enzymes, minerals and other nutrients from the colon, together with the friendly bacteria which are vital for good digestion. This can increase the risk of a mineral imbalance. On the other hand, high colonics don't serve the all-important reason for the use of coffee enemas, namely the opening of the bile ducts, which helps the liver to release toxins and cleanse itself. **On no account should anyone make the mistake of thinking that high colonics are interchangeable with coffee enemas.**

We have presented the history and theoretical background. Now let us the practicalities.

The Basics and How to Use Them

The basic components of the coffee enema are the following:

- Organic, medium or light roast drip-grind coffee

- Filtered, or if from a fluoridated source, distilled water

- Enema equipment

The equipment must be carefully chosen, as not all products on the market are suitable. The earliest type—the combination syringe—is a rubber hot-water bottle, complete with appropriate tubing and rectal or vaginal tip. This works well for occasional use or travel but it is difficult to clean. Other rubber bags, not "combination syringes," have a much wider opening, which makes them easier to clean. However, they don't stand up well to constant use.

Most popular among Gerson patients is the plastic bucket, which has an easy-to-read register of ounces. This shows how much of the coffee the patient has introduced into the rectum. The bucket is easy to clean and has only one drawback: if dropped or cleaned too vigorously, it can break and must be replaced.

That risk is avoided by choosing a stainless steel bucket, now available at the relatively cheap price of about $30, including the needed attachments. It is unbreakable and easy to clean, even with very hot water, which shouldn't be used with the plastic bucket. The rubber tubing needs to be replaced occasionally. The only disadvantage of this type is that, not being transparent, one cannot check how far the enema process has progressed.

The standard mixture for one enema consists of 3 rounded tablespoons of organic, medium or light roast drip-grind coffee and 32 ounces of filtered or distilled water. The procedure is to bring the water to a boil, add the coffee, let it boil for 3 minutes, then turn down the heat and let it simmer (covered) for 15 minutes. Let it cool, then strain it through a cloth-lined strainer. (A piece of clean, white linen or nylon can be used.) Check the amount left after straining and replace the water that has boiled away to restore it to 1 quart.

For patients on the therapy, it is best to prepare the whole day's requirement at once rather than cooking each portion separately every 4 hours. In other words, a coffee concentrate is produced, saving much time and effort. Take a pot which holds at least 3 quarts, put in about 2 quarts of filtered or distilled water, bring it to a boil and add 15 rounded tablespoons of coffee, which will be enough for five enemas, then proceed as above. After straining the liquid, take five 1-quart jars or juice bottles, pour the same amount of the concentrate into each, then add enough water to make up the volume to 8 ounces of concentrate.

The standard mixture for one enema (i.e., 8 ounces of coffee concentrate and 24 ounces of water, making a total of 32 ounces) has to be warmed to body temperature and poured into the enema bucket, having first clamped the tube shut to stop the liquid from running out. Before starting the enema, a small amount of the solution should be released to clear the tube of air. It is a good idea to eat a small piece of fruit to get the digestive system going, especially before the first morning enema. This will provide a little glucose to raise the low blood sugar after a night's sleep.

The more relaxed the patient is, the easier the enema experience will be. That requires comfort. Unless a couch or folding camp bed is available, an enema "nest" is made on the bathroom floor, with a large, soft towel or blanket as its base, covered with an enema mat or a soft polyester shower curtain for accidental leaks or spillage and a pillow or cushion for the head. **The bucket is placed at approximately 18 inches above the body, hanging from a hook or standing on a stool. The coffee should not flow in too fast or with too much pressure.** About 2 inches of the tube's tip is lubricated with Vaseline® and gently inserted some 8 to 10 inches into the anus, and the clamp on the tube is released to let the coffee flow in. **The patient lies on his or her right side with legs pulled up in the fetal position, relaxed and breathing deeply. When all the coffee is absorbed, it should be held in for 12 to 15 minutes, before evacuating.**

Many patients enjoy the relaxed comfort of enema time—**"upside-down coffee,"** as some call it—and use it to listen to soothing music, to meditate or to read. One young lady, recovering from a brain tumor on the Gerson program over some two years, first read all the main classics, then switched to philosophy, followed by mathematics, and subsequently became so well read that she won a top scholarship! She also made a full recovery.

How Many? How Often?

Most patients with bone and joint diseases can do with two or three enemas a day. Unless they are seriously ill with kidney problems, nonhealing skin lesions and sores or gangrene of the extremities, they can use a somewhat easier therapy. If the problems are more severe, they will do better, respond faster and heal with a stricter approach.

In such cases, more juices (eight to 10 glasses a day) and more enemas (four to five a day) are suggested. It is important to remember that juice intake has to be adjusted to enema use since enemas tend to flush out minerals from the large intestine (causing electrolyte imbalance) unless these are replenished with the intake of juices, high in minerals.

Also remember that coffee enemas do not interfere with the normal activity of the colon, producing daily bowel movements. Occasionally, patients worry about that but their fears are groundless. Once the liver and the digestive system are fully restored, normal elimination takes over, even in those who had previously suffered from constipation.

Possible Problems

Many patients learn the enema routine without difficulty and enjoy the feeling of lightness and added energy yielded by the practice. Others, however, experience difficulties, which need to be addressed. Some of the problems that may arise are listed below.

Patients may arrive at the hospital with a massive accumulation of stool in their colon, caused by the use of heavy pain-killing drugs, including morphine. These tend to paralyze peristalsis (the alternate contraction and relaxation of the intestine, by which the contents are propelled onward), causing severe constipation. As a result, these patients are unable to take in a quart (32 ounces) of the coffee solution, let alone hold it in. The answer for them is to take whatever amount they can comfortably accommodate, stop and hold this as long as possible (even if only for a few minutes), then release and take the remaining coffee solution. Again, hold it and release after 12 to 15 minutes. As a rule, after two or three days, when the colon has been cleared of old accumulations, the whole enemas can be taken and held without difficulty.

Some patients may suffer from gas retention, which stops the enema from getting into the colon. When that happens, a small amount—say 6 to 10 ounces—of the coffee can be infused, after which the bucket is lowered to the patient's level, allowing the coffee to flow back into the bucket. This often releases the gas, causing some "bubbling" in the bucket. The bucket is then raised again and, after the clearing of the gas, the enema can continue more easily.

The patient is supposed to take the enema lying on his or her right side in order to help the coffee solution get into the transverse colon from the descending colon. However, as a result of surgery or arthritis, the right side may be painful. In such a case, the patient can lie on his or her back, with their legs pulled up, and proceed from that position.

If a patient suffers from severe irritation of the colon, a small portion of the coffee concentrate, say 2 to 4 ounces, can be diluted with chamomile tea instead of water. The smaller amount of coffee will still help to detoxify the liver while the chamomile tea soothes the colon. There is no time limit for the use of chamomile tea. **In the case of severe diarrhea, an enema of chamomile tea only is used for gentle morning and evening cleansing.**

To prepare chamomile tea, put 1 ounce of the dried flower heads into a glass dish, add 1 pint of boiling water, cover the dish and let it stand in a warm place to infuse for 15 minutes. Strain, cool and store it in a stoppered bottle for a maximum of three days. Increase amounts in the above proportion as required. Chamomile is one of the herbs most used in the Gerson Therapy, both as an enema component and as an herbal drink.

Sometimes a patient has been doing enemas for the first few days of the treatment without a problem, but suddenly he or she cannot get more than 8 to 12 ounces into the colon. This may be a symptom of a healing reaction or flare-up, and the solution is to take what is possible, release it and take the rest. Even if the coffee solution has to be infused in three small amounts, it doesn't matter.

Flare-ups are dealt with in detail in Chapter 14, "Understanding Healing Reactions," p. 127. In brief, they occur when so much bile is released that the intestine is unable to contain it all. The bile then overflows and backs up into the stomach. Since the stomach needs to be acid in order to hold and digest food, the highly alkaline bile produces enormous discomfort; the stomach cannot hold food or liquid and the patient vomits. In itself, this type of flare-up is welcome because it clears out a lot of toxic bile but, in the process, the stomach membrane becomes irritated and needs instant relief. **To do that, the patient needs to drink as much peppermint tea and oatmeal gruel (see Chapter 14) as possible.** At the same time, the coffee enemas are reduced since they are causing the heavy flow of bile. The correct order for the next two to three days is two chamomile enemas and only one coffee enema a day, until the nausea and vomiting clear up. Then the regular schedule can be resumed.

During the flare-up, if the patient vomits and also has diarrhea, the body loses a lot of fluid, so dehydration must be prevented.

One way is to use more chamomile enemas instead of coffee. Also, the apple/carrot and green juices can be used as rectal implants. The regular 8-ounce dose of juice is warmed to body temperature by placing the glass in a warm water bath (not on the stove and without diluting it) and gently infused into the rectum. **This is not an enema and the patient should hold it until the liquid is absorbed.** That may not take more than 10 to 15 minutes of lying still in bed. These infusions can be used with all the juices (except orange and grapefruit) every hour, instead of having them as drinks—particularly valuable at times when, during the flare-up, the patient cannot even bear to look at a juice, let alone drink it.

Another problem occurs when the patient takes in the full 32 ounces of coffee solution but, after 12 minutes, is unable to release it. When that happens, the usual reaction is to take another enema, expecting it to push out the first lot, but that doesn't happen and the patient tends to panic. The reason for the blockage is that the colon spasms, cramps and doesn't release the liquid. Of course, there is no danger in this—the colon could actually hold up to 5 quarts—but that is not the point. If the trouble is caused by cramping, the patient needs to lie down on his or her side, with a warm water bottle on their stomach, and try to relax. If the situation lasts a little longer, including the time for the next enema, it helps to put 2 tablespoons of the regular potassium compound (see Chapter 13, "Medications," p. 121) into each enema for a few days. This will help to release cramps and/or spasms.

Please note: **Do not use this method for more than two to three days to avoid irritating the rectum and the colon.**

It is only when they are on the regular enema routine that patients realize how much waste material their bodies have stored over many years. Once the organism gets a go-ahead in the direction of self-cleansing, it does release a variety of strange, disturbing accumulations which appear in the enema returns, including a wide range of parasites. Experts claim that some 85% of us harbor parasites in our colon, which are best expelled. So the message is not to panic **if the enema returns contain unusual substances; they prove that detoxification and cleansing is progressing well.**

Cleaning the Equipment

Like all other tools of the Gerson program, the enema bucket has to be kept clean. Since the anus, rectum and colon are not sterile, the equipment need not be sterilized. After each use, the bucket has to be rinsed with hot, soapy water, running it through the tube as well, and then rinsed again thoroughly to remove the soap. **Two or three times a week, it is wise to put a cup of 3% hydrogen peroxide (from the super-**

market or drug store) into the bucket with the clamp closed and let it stand overnight to kill any germs or impurities. Rinse it out before the first use in the morning.

CAUTION

If you keep the plastic tube attached to the bucket, it will eventually become loose and even slip off, treating you to an unwanted coffee shower. Check the fit frequently and, if necessary, cut an inch or so from the loosened end of the tube and replace the tight part. You can prevent accidents by removing the plastic tube every time before running hot water through the bucket, so that it shrinks back to its original size and remains tightly in position.

CHAPTER 12 REFERENCES

1. M. Gerson, *A Cancer Therapy: Results of Fifty Cases and The Cure of Advanced Cancer by Diet Therapy: A Summary of Thirty Years of Clinical Experimentation,* 6th ed. (San Diego, CA: Gerson Institute, 1999).
2. Peter Lechner, MD, "Dietary Regime to be Used in Oncological Postoperative Care," Proceedings of the Oesterreicher Gesellschaft fur Chirurgie (Jun. 21-23, 1984).

CHAPTER 13

Medications

F or the general public, "medications" normally mean drugs, used in allopathic medicine in the treatment of disease. In acute cases and emergencies, many drugs are life saving and highly valuable. However, when it comes to chronic conditions, as a rule, the synthetic drugs, which are alien to the body, can merely alleviate (i.e., suppress) symptoms without dealing with the basic cause. This process is often accompanied by severe side effects, which may require more drugs to control.

The medications used in the Gerson Therapy belong to a totally different category. Far from being drugs, they are nutritional supplements consisting of natural substances present in, and needed for, the normal functioning of the various body systems. Being natural, they have no damaging side effects. Their purpose is to make up for the deficiencies of the sick body until it recovers sufficiently to cover all its needs. These substances are so pure that, even if they are incorrectly used by mistake or are in excessive or insufficient doses, they do no harm—with the exception of the thyroid/iodine supplementation, which must be correctly adjusted.

Let us take them one by one and explore their purpose.

Potassium Compound

Dr. Gerson found that the basic problem in all chronic degenerative diseases is the loss of potassium from, and the penetration of sodium into, the cells, now known as the tissue damage syndrome. The average diet in most countries, especially in the developed world, contains far too much salt (sodium), which eventually causes the breakdown of the healthy balance within the body.[1] To correct this, Dr. Gerson added a large amount of potassium (a 10% solution of three potassium salts) to the already potassium-rich, organic vegetarian diet, and observed that this enabled the sick body to release the excess sodium, together with edema, while also reducing high blood pressure and, in most cases, pain.

To prepare the compound, 100 grams of three ready-mixed potassium salts are dissolved in 1 quart of distilled water and stored in a dark glass bottle, or in a clear one kept inside a large brown or black paper bag, to keep out all light. On the full intensive therapy, 4 teaspoons of the potassium compound are added to 10 of the freshly prepared fruit and/or vegetable juices. This dosage is reduced after three to four weeks to 2 teaspoons in each of 10 juices.

In seriously ill patients, it takes many months, even one to two years, to restore normal potassium content to the essential organs. The serum potassium level, as shown in the blood test result, does not reflect the potassium status of the cell. Low serum potassium values may signify healing because the depleted tissues are reabsorbing potassium, while high figures may be found in failures because the tissues lose it.

Thyroid and Lugol's Solution

It is a fact—known since Dr. Gerson's day—that most chronically ill patients are suffering from a low basal metabolism.[2] Much of the problem is caused by the chlorine,[3] widely used in the purification of the water supply and, worse still, by fluoride.[4] **Both remove iodine from the thyroid gland,** thus reducing its ability to function properly. The thyroid gland regulates the metabolic rate of the organism, acting as its thermostat, being capable of raising temperature and producing fever. It also affects the immune system as well as the proper functioning of all hormone systems. In high blood pressure caused by atherosclerosis, low metabolism slows the burning of fats, encouraging narrowing of the arteries.

When thyroid and iodine in the form of 1/2 strength Lugol's solution are added to the patient's intake, the immune system becomes reactivated and healing can begin. The patient can start with the doses outlined in Table 15-1, "Schedule for Nonmalignant Patients" in Chapter 15, "The Gerson Therapy for Nonmalignant Diseases," p. 134, and be monitored by a trained Gerson doctor. Thyroid hormone levels may also determined by the patient directly using blood chemistry tests ordered from Direct Labs (www.directlabs.com). This confidential laboratory testing service offers a private and secure online portal where you can order your test and retrieve your results at a very reasonable cost.

The process is simple:

1. Contact Direct Labs to open an account, complete the necessary authorizations and order your test.
2. You will then choose a local laboratory that will draw your blood.
3. In 24 to 48 hours, you will receive an email letting you know that you may log in to your account to view or print your results.

Niacin

Niacin (common name for nicotinic acid, or vitamin B_3) assists in the digestion of protein and helps to open capillary circulation, thus bringing freshly oxygenated blood (from the constant intake of fresh juices) to all body tissues. By improving circulation, it also works to reduce ascites (an abdominal edema where excess water is retained in the abdomen) and pain. The dosage is a 50 mg tablet five times daily, taken during meals. This medication often causes the well-known "niacin flush," a temporary reddening of the face and upper chest area, with some itching. This is totally harmless and passes quickly. (**Do not**

switch to nonflushing niacin; it is ineffective.) Niacin should be discontinued during women's periods or in case of bleeding of any kind.

Liver Capsules

The severely toxic and damaged liver needs maximum assistance to improve its vital functions. The therapy provides this help in the form of liver capsules containing dried, defatted, powdered liver from healthy animals. Two capsules of liver powder are given three times a day with carrot-only juice. According to Dr. Virginia Livingston,[5] the combination of dry liver powder with carrot juice produces abscisic acid, a precursor of vitamin A.

Crude Liver Injections with B_{12} Supplement

Since most chronic disease patients are also anemic (a condition that develops when your blood lacks enough healthy red blood cells), additional vitamin B_{12} is needed to help restore the hemoglobin content of the blood, promoting the formation and maturation of red blood cells. It works against different types of anemia and even against degenerative changes in the spinal cord. As seen in animal experiments, this vitamin is able to restore a wide range of tissues damaged by age, chronic illness, surgery, degenerative diseases or various kinds of poisoning. Intramuscular liver extract (3 cc) with added 50 mcg of B_{12}—a tiny amount, a 20th of 1 cc—is given every other day. The frequency is reduced as patient shows recovery.

Pancreatin

This is an extract of various pancreatic digestive enzymes, normally needed to digest fats, proteins and sugar. Gerson patients don't consume those substances; however, these enzymes are vitally important in the digestion and elimination of atherosclerosis. The dosage is 3 tablets of 325 mg each four times a day—one after each meal, plus an additional dose in mid-afternoon.

Acidol Pepsin

This can be used if the patient has a poor appetite since it helps with digestion. **No acidol is given in cases of acid reflux, stomach ulcers, or other irritation of the stomach.**

Flaxseed Oil

Also known as food-grade linseed oil, this contains both essential fatty acids—linoleic acid and linolenic acid—and is particularly rich in the Omega-3 series, as discovered by Johanna Budwig, PhD.[6] The therapeutic effects of flaxseed oil include the following:

- It attracts oxygen at the cell membrane and transports oxygen into the cell.

- It is able to detoxify fat-soluble toxins and helps to dissolve and remove plaque.

- It is a carrier of vitamin A, which is important for the immune system.

- It removes excess cholesterol, an important function, since patients' cholesterol levels sometimes rise during the initial stages of the therapy.

The dose is 2 tablespoons daily for the first month, then 1 tablespoon daily for the rest of the treatment (limited, similar to medications, and reduced to 1 tablespoon daily after 30 days).

Coenzyme Q10

Recently added to the protocol, this coenzyme is valuable in replacing some of the nutrients that were available in the discontinued raw liver juice. It must be administered cautiously at first, since some patients are hypersensitive to this substance. To start, the dose is 50 mg daily for five to seven days, then increased to 100 mg per day, to reach 500 to 600 mg daily.

CHAPTER 13 REFERENCES

1. Freeman Widener Cope, *Physiological Chemistry and Physics* 10 (5) (1978).
2. Kathy Page, "Hypothyroidism and Cancer," supplementary memorandum, UK Parliament Select Committee on Science and Technology (June 2000).
3. Joseph M. Price, *Coronaries, cholesterol, chlorine* (Salem, MA: Pyramid Books, 1971).
4. P. M. Galetti and G. Joyet, "Effect of fluorine on thyroidal iodine metabolism in hyperthyroidism," *Journal of Clinical Endocrinology and Metabolism* 18 (10) (October 1958): 1102-10.
5. Personal communication from Dr. Livingston to Charlotte Gerson (February 1977).
6. Johanna Budwig, PhD, *Flax Oil As a True Aid Against Arthritis Heart Infarction Cancer and Other Diseases,* 3d ed. (Ferndale, WA: Apple Publishing, December 1994).

CHAPTER 14

Understanding Healing Reactions

Healing reactions, also known as flare-ups, are an essential part of the Gerson Therapy. It is important that patients understand their nature and function before embarking on the full treatment, since healing reactions are somewhat paradoxical experiences: although they can produce a number of unpleasant symptoms, they should be welcomed as evidence that the therapy has kicked in and is working well.

Let's see how and when this necessary process is likely to begin. As a rule, after the first few days on the full Gerson program, the patients feel better. Naturally they are greatly encouraged. That is the moment to remind them that a healing reaction may be on the way and to explain how it is going to promote detoxification. Without proper preparation, the sudden shift is hard to bear!

Arthritic patients are usually less severely ill than those with diabetes, high blood pressure, cancer, etc., due to the highly toxic medications the latter are taking. Nevertheless, both patients and doctors need to understand that the entire public eating the "standard American diet" has accumulated a level of toxicity, no matter what their diagnosis or disease—even if they are not sick! Therefore, as the Gerson Therapy begins to work, the fatty tissue dissolves and releases toxic materials the body has stored there!

In addition, when the reactions start, the calcium deposits in the arteries (atherosclerosis) are released into the bloodstream and could cause clots. This does not happen when the therapy is faithfully practiced. The regimen should not be changed during such a flare-up or "healing reaction." This protects the patient and we have observed no sudden clotting (heart attacks or strokes). No blood-thinning drugs should be needed.

Again, the patient must be prepared for these reactions, which may be accompanied by toxic stools, lack of appetite and even aversion to food or drink, especially to the green juices. There can also be more gas than usual, plus difficulties with the coffee enemas (due to increased toxic pressure from the liver). **Without advance warning, the patients may feel that their condition is worsening.**

The first flare-up is usually relatively short, since the body is not yet able to carry out serious healing in its weakened condition and is only just beginning to respond. Even that early start can produce impressive results. The body begins to heal old injuries, fractures, lumpy scars and serious conditions, including long-standing high blood pressure and age-onset diabetes. **This process cannot be held back or stopped since the body is not able to heal selectively!** In other words, it does not only heal the present life-threatening disease but also clears up all other damage, whether old or new. That is what the totality of the Gerson Therapy means. Thanks to it, patients have overcome allergies, long-term migraines, arthritis, fibromyalgia and other conditions that have troubled them for any length of time.

How do patients react to a flare-up? Only a general answer can be given based on the reactions of a majority of cases. Since each person is different and has a different medical past with different damages to the body, each healing reaction is also different. It is also impossible to give an exact answer to patients who wish to know how long a flare-up will last. In many cases, the first reaction is mild and only lasts from a few hours to a day or two. The second one is normally longer and somewhat heavier, since the body and its immune system have, to some extent, been detoxified, strengthened with the enzymes and nutrients contained in the raw juices and supported by the medication. As a result, it is able to respond more powerfully.

What should one do for the patient in a flare-up who is unwell, upset and dismayed? One should not stop the therapy and give no coffee enemas or juices, for doing so would drastically stop the healing process, yet we must help the patient to endure the discomforts of the flare-ups. Here are the best ways:

Nausea

If, despite the nausea, the patient is able to drink the juices, by all means continue to provide them. If he or she develops a severe aversion to the green juice, warm it gently (undiluted) to body temperature by standing the container in a warm water bath, pour the juice into the enema bucket and infuse it rectally as a retention implant. **This is not an enema and should not be expelled.**

The patient should lie comfortably in bed, with legs pulled up in the fetal position, and allow the juice to be absorbed. Patients who are temporarily unable to drink any juices can have them administered rectally (all except the orange juice) and should be encouraged to drink warm oatmeal gruel and plenty of peppermint tea, partly to settle the stomach and also to supply the necessary liquids which would normally be provided by the juices.

To prepare oatmeal gruel, place 1 ounce of oats and 5 ounces of water into a pot and bring to a boil. Let it simmer for 10 to 15 minutes, then strain through a fine tea strainer to remove all solids. Press the oats as far as possible through the strainer in order to obtain a liquid somewhat denser than water. Drink while warm.

For patients severely sensitive to juices during a flare-up, 2 ounces of gruel can be poured into a glass and topped with no more than 6 ounces of juice.

Peppermint tea helps to relieve nausea, digestive discomfort and gas. Peppermint or spearmint is easy to grow in the backyard and spreads quickly. A heaped tablespoon of fresh leaves makes one cup of tea; add boiling distilled water, cover and let it steep for 12 to 15 minutes, then strain. If you use tea bags, make sure they are organic. One tea bag easily makes two cups. If you buy loose leaves, which is preferable, put a table-spoon of leaves in the pot, pour 2 cups of boiling distilled water over them, and proceed as above.

It is a good idea to leave peppermint tea in a thermos on the patient's bedside table, in case he or she wakes up thirsty at night.

Controlling Diarrhea

- Stop all juices. Give the patient frequent cups of peppermint tea, at least 5 or 6 daily. Add 1/8 teaspoon of potassium gluco-nate powder (**not the potassium compound**) in every cup.

- Food should consist of oatmeal 3 times per day, with brown sugar (no honey) and applesauce.

- Suspend coffee enemas. Use only chamomile tea enemas 2-3 times per day.

- Restart coffee enemas when condition improves. It is best to restart enemas using camomile tea to dilute the coffee concentrate.

- As the intestinal tract calms down, gradually start juices. Place 2-3 ounces of oatmeal gruel into each cup, then add 5-6 ounces of juice. Do not add any medication. Avoid salads for 1-2 days. Continue oatmeal with applesauce.

- When juices are tolerated, add medication.

- Gradually reduce peppermint tea.

- Appetite may be temporarily reduced but will return later. Meanwhile, raw foods are better tolerated than cooked dishes. However, if patient prefers, he/she can use soup, potatoes (without eating the skin) and some cooked, soft vegetables.

- You can give 2 charcoal tablets, ground up in tea, after each loose bowel movement. This helps to absorb and reduce gas or other discomfort.

- If diarrhea lasts for more than 3 days, the stool specimen should be tested. However, diarrhea is mostly one of the symptoms of the healing reaction.

Depression

Dr. Gerson notes[1] that it is not unusual for the patient to be depressed, temporarily during a flare-up. Such emotional outbursts run parallel with the body's attempts to detoxify: **remember the mind and body are connected and cannot be separated.**

Often, an extra enema helps to ease the upheaval. The patient may even pick a fight with the caregiver for no obvious reason. This is less surprising if we consider the metabolic fact that aggression produces extra adrenalin, which makes the person actually feel better! The caregiver should not be hurt by any unwarranted attacks or accusations. The patient cannot control these outbursts and usually regrets them afterwards. Again, a coffee enema can clear the problem. This part of the healing reaction should be seen as a psychological cleansing. Once the flare-up is over, the patient will again be optimistic and forward-looking.

CHAPTER 14 REFERENCE

1. M. Gerson, *A Cancer Therapy: Results of Fifty Cases and The Cure of Advanced Cancer by Diet Therapy: A Summary of Thirty Years of Clinical Experimentation,* 6th ed. (San Diego, CA: Gerson Institute, 1999), pp. 201-202.

CHAPTER 15

The Gerson Therapy for Nonmalignant Diseases

From his long clinical practice, Dr. Gerson was able to establish that a patient suffering from a nonmalignant disease had a sick, damaged liver, while the liver of someone with a malignancy was severely toxic (poisoned). Based on this difference, he adjusted the treatment accordingly, creating a less-intensive therapy for nonmalignant conditions. At the same time, he specified that, if patients in the latter category followed a stricter protocol closely resembling the full intensive therapy, they recovered faster.

The less-intensive therapy is less demanding and easier to follow, so that patients on this regime can continue working. This is a great advantage since most people depend on their earned income and cannot leave their jobs for any length of time. Table 15-1 is a typical hour-by-hour schedule for patients on the less-intensive therapy.

Note for Table 15-1

- Make yourself a blank schedule to be filled in later as the medications change and the frequency of enemas is reduced.

Table 15-1
SCHEDULE FOR NONMALIGNANT PATIENT

	Enema	Meal	Flaxseed Oil (tbsp.)	Acidol Pepsin Capsules	Juice	Potassium Compound (tsp.)	Lugol's Solution (1/2 Strength) (drops)	Thyroid (gr.)	Niacin (mg.)	Liver Capsules	Pancreatin Tablets	Liver and B₁₂ Injection
8:00 a.m.		Breakfast		2	Orange	2	1	1	50	2	3	
9:00 a.m.	Coffee				Green	2						
10:00 a.m.					Carrot/apple	2			50			
11:00 a.m.					Carrot					2		Every 2nd day
12:00 p.m.					Green	2						
1:00 p.m.		Lunch	1	2	Carrot/apple	2	1	1	50		3	
2:00 p.m.	Coffee				Green	2						
5:00 p.m.					Carrot/apple	2			50		3	
6:00 p.m.	Coffee				Green	2						
7:00 p.m.		Dinner	1	2	Carrot/apple	2	1	1	50	2	3	

It is difficult to specify the amount of time it may take for patients to reduce the intensity of the treatment. It depends on the degree of damage, their ability to heal, their age, encouragement and help in the home, and possible psychological factors. Often, the patient knows when the time is right. Nonetheless, it is important not to discontinue the treatment too soon or too abruptly. Serious problems could result.

CHAPTER 16

Things to Remember

I n this chapter, we present a number of miscellaneous items in support of your efforts to improve and protect your health. Knowledge is power, and the emergence of the so-called "expert patient" around the world is a sure sign that more and more people are willing to take responsibility for their health and well-being. No doubt you are one of them. We hope you will find the following information useful.

Complementary Therapies

These days, there is a bewildering array of complementary treatments offered and the question arises whether Gerson patients should use any of these. The simple answer is that anything which promotes healing and does not clash with the requirements of the therapy is permissible and potentially helpful. However, there is little margin for error, so let us review which techniques are safe to use.

Reflexology or Zone Therapy

This dates back to ancient Egypt, China and India. **It is based on the principle that the feet and hands are a mirror image of the body** and that, by applying pressure to certain points—especially on the feet—corresponding parts of the body are affected. The purpose of the treatment is to break up congestion, blockages and patterns of stress and restore homeostasis, the body's internal equilibrium. Reflexology does not claim to diagnose or cure, but it has a good record of improving general well-being.

Reiki

 This is a Japanese technique for stress reduction and relaxation that promotes healing. **Its practitioners claim that there is an invisible life-force energy that flows through us and keeps us alive.** If this energy becomes low, we fall sick and suffer from stress. In order to heal, the Reiki master channels the energy through his or her hands into the patient's body. There is no need for massage, only for very gentle touch. Although the patient feels very little, the treatment is truly holistic, affecting body, emotions, mind and spirit. Because of its nonspecific nature, Reiki is able to help in any disease and works well with other medical or therapeutic techniques. The word itself consists of two parts: *Rei* means higher power and *Ki* stands for life-force energy, so the implication is that Reiki is a spiritually guided way of restoring universal life-force energy in those who need it.

Acupuncture

This originated in China some 2,000 years ago and has been known and increasingly practiced in the United States since 1971. Its essence is the stimulation of certain anatomical points on the body by penetrating the skin with thin metal nee- dles and manipulating them by hand or electrical means. This is claimed to regulate the nervous system, activate the body's own painkilling biochemicals and strengthen the immune system. Acupuncture has a proven record of good pain control and of hastening recovery from surgery. It can impart a sense of well-being and boosts depleted energy. Acupuncture needles, which cause minimal pain, were approved by the Food and Drug Administration for use by licensed practitioners in 1996.[1] Today, this ancient technique is used in the United States by thousands of physicians, dentists and other practitioners for the prevention or relief of pain.

Yoga

 Yoga first emerged in India some 5,000 years ago. It has several varieties, including hatha yoga, a physical discipline consisting mainly of stretching and breathing exercises, which has grown in popularity in the West since the mid-20th century. Being noncompetitive, gentle and accessible to people of all ages and levels of ability, yoga is an ideal exercise for Gerson patients who wish to improve their flexibility, stamina and muscle tone. Yoga postures, known as asanas, help to achieve balance and poise. The breathing exercises are soothing and relaxing and increase the supply of oxygen to the organism.

Chi Gung

Ancient Chinese teachings advise that vital life force energy—also known as "chi"—flows through your body in specific channels or rivers called "meridians." When the meridians are open and flowing properly, the body is strong and healthy. When the meridians are obstructed or chi flow is blocked, health wanes, resulting in sickness and disease.

Interestingly, there is some agreement between Dr. Gerson's reasons for poor health and the principles of chi gung (pronounced *chee-gung*) regarding blocked chi flow. They both may result from poor diet, toxicity, a sedentary lifestyle and stress.

While chi gung is relatively new in Western society, quite a bit of research has been done in the East supporting its health benefits. Millions of people around the world practice chi gung every day because they say it makes them healthier, boosts their energy and helps them feel better.

Practitioners of chi gung learn to strengthen their life-force energy and open their meridians by combining slow body movements with deep-breathing techniques and mental visualizations that cause their chi to move throughout the body. Chi gung is an excellent exercise for Gerson patients of all ages as it is done in a relaxed manner and creates no pain or stress in your body.

CHAPTER 16 REFERENCE

1. "Get the Facts: Acupuncture," National Center for Complementary and Alternative Medicine (http://nccam.nih.gov/health/acupuncture).

CHAPTER 17

Watch Out: Pitfalls Ahead!

As humans, we can make mistakes in any area of life—but when seriously ill people undertake a potentially life-saving program, such as the Gerson Therapy, even a minor blunder or oversight could cause a setback. This way of healing demands a total transformation—not only of lifestyle but also of how the patients understand the principles of sickness, health and healing, and how they respond to their bodies' needs. This understanding is all the more important because the therapy forbids a great many things that are normal parts of the Western lifestyle, and patients need to know the reason behind the strictures in order to accept them wholeheartedly.

There is also the matter of observing the rules of the therapy, even without an authority figure to check or chide the patient as there would be in a conventional medical setting. **It takes maturity and inner strength to be one's own supervisor and stay on the straight and narrow path, but the rewards are enormous and make it all more than worthwhile.**

Save Up Your Energy!

Let's take a close look at the possible mistakes, temptations and trip-wires that a patient is likely to encounter, especially in the early stages of the Gerson protocol. Ironically, the first pitfall is the great improvement in the patient's condition that sets in during the first few weeks on the full therapy, especially if these are spent at the Gerson clinic in Mexico.

When such patients return home—and this holds true especially for women—they look and feel better and are often free from pain, so the family assumes that they can once again rely on the patients to take up all "normal" duties and serve them.

- This is a particularly heavy burden on the wife/mother, who probably feels guilty anyway for "letting down" the family by being ill and having very real needs of her own; guilt may drive her back into her normal routine.

- Male patients normally have a more relaxed attitude on coming home, but even they want to start to work, exercise or deal with chores around the house.

- **Neither behavior is acceptable.**

As stated before, patients need a great deal of rest. Their bodies are working hard to detoxify and heal, and that is more important than any domestic activity. Actually, in most cases, although patients look remarkably better, they do feel tired and even weak for the first two to three months of the therapy, unable to indulge in much activity. Instead of listening to their bodies' message, some patients actually force themselves to be up, make their own food and juice (a six- to eight-hour daily job!) and exhaust themselves. That is a serious mistake.

A similar problem arises, three to four months into the therapy, when the initial tiredness goes and energy returns to such an extent that patients feel virtually normal. They want to be fully active again and make up for "lost time."

Women launch themselves into major housecleaning by washing curtains, scrubbing floors and attacking mountains of ironing; men clear out the garage and, according to the season, either shovel snow or cut the lawn, or even repair the roof, just to prove that they are fully functioning once more. The urge is understandable but must be resisted to avoid a sudden downturn. **Superficial improvements (e.g., increased energy) do not equal healing.** Rest and more rest are still essential to avoid a sudden downturn.

One of Dr. Gerson's important rules was that patients should be in bed no later than 10 p.m.—not reading or watching television or listening to the radio—but sleeping, if possible, or at least at complete rest. The time before midnight is particularly valuable for the body's self-repairing and restoring work and must not be curtailed.

Bending the Rules

Admittedly, the dietary rules of the Gerson Therapy are pretty strict and, while most patients quickly get used to them, there are some who long for their now-forbidden favorite foods (never mind that those had probably contributed to their health breakdown!). **These patients tend to think that surely having a "little extra" on the side every now and then can't possibly do much harm, and would even raise their morale and improve their mood.**

This is wrong on all counts. First of all, how much is "a little" and how often is "every now and then"? Furthermore, once the strict adherence to the protocol is broken, it's easy and tempting to break it again ... and again. Also consider that, since in this treatment the body receives instructions and messages via precisely calculated nutrients, each of which affects all the others, to disturb the process with occasional additions of salty, fatty, chemical-laden junk food sounds like a disastrous idea.

Often, it is not the patient but well-meaning visitors—friends and relatives—who suggest breaking the diet and having "a nice big steak to build you up!" They are the ones who question how a grown person can survive, let alone heal, on all that "rabbit food" and, even if the patient manages to ignore their advice, a certain irritation ensues. **Please remember that people who criticize the Gerson protocol, including** otherwise helpful and well-meaning health professionals, do so out of ignorance and incomprehension and, for that reason, can be safely ignored. It's best to ask your visitors and friends to please respect your choice of treatment and support and encourage you—or else leave you alone. Ask those who suggest changes to the therapy, "How many patients have you healed with your advice?"

Being Firm with Friendly Doctors

A friendly allopathic doctor willing to support a Gerson patient is a great asset if he or she agrees to prescribe the necessary blood tests and urinalyses. The problem arises when he or she reads the test results. If any item is out of the normal range, the doctor suggests that the patient take some drug or medication "to bring it to the normal level." That, too, can be a serious mistake. The abnormal value will clear up on the Gerson Therapy, but allopathic drugs can cause damage.

For example, we know of a doctor who noticed a somewhat low iron level in the patient's blood and prescribed an iron medication. The trouble is that iron supplements are toxic,[1] which automatically rules them out for Gerson patients. In time, with all the green juices, liver medication and vitamin B_{12}, the blood readings will return to normal without drugs.

Flare-Ups and Mood Swings

Healing reactions or so-called flare-ups are regular events on the Gerson Therapy. (See Chapter 14, "Understanding Healing Reactions," p. 127.) These episodes can be frighteningly intense; at the same time, the patient may also suffer from depression and a black mood. If the family panics, the patient may end up in the emergency room of the nearest hospital, where the doctors are kind and concerned and give the patient a shot or a pill to stop the symptoms. Unfortunately, they also stop the healing, which has caused serious problems in some cases. **The fact is that the average allopathic doctor has probably never heard of a healing reaction, does not understand its symptoms and function and**

therefore can't be expected to handle it correctly. The proper way to deal with a flare-up is clearly set out in Chapter 14 and should be followed closely.

Psychological problems and mood swings are dealt with fully. Here, we only want to acknowledge the power of occasional fits of negativity, when the patient not only feels physically unwell—with nausea, sweating, headache, horror of food and juices and possibly fever—but is also mentally and emotionally crushed. The toxins cruising through the central nervous system and the brain are to blame, but all the patient feels is an urgent wish to stop the therapy, break out of all the restrictions and run away. This is a passing phase. It is wise to find out about it in advance so that, when it arrives, the patient is more or less prepared and snaps out of it faster.

Water Warning

Don't underestimate the importance of ensuring the purity of all the water used in your home. The worst offender is fluoride, so make sure that your water supply is free from this harmful chemical. If it is not, you must take special precautions. **Unlike chlorine, fluoride is not eliminated by boiling the water! The only way to get rid of it is by distillation. (See Chapter 8, "The Gerson Household," p. 79.)**

However, fluoride is also present in the water used for the daily shower. Although a shower needn't take many minutes, even brief exposure to warm water opens the pores, so that any undesirable component in the water gets quickly absorbed. There are two solutions to this problem:

- Take a sponge bath, instead of a shower, in a gallon of warmed distilled water poured into a basin or sink.

- Install a camping shower in the bathroom and fill it with warmed distilled water. Full description, various models and prices of this appliance are available on the Internet.

Mind What You Read

Knowledge is power and the well-informed patient is likely to make the right choices. However, the big and growing range of so-called health books and diet bibles is a dangerous area full of contradictory theories and advice. Open-minded patients keen to learn new things read as many health books as they can find and end up confused. Although most nutritional methods are at least in part based on the Gerson Therapy, none is complete or free from its author's prejudices and subjective ideas.

If you have decided to use the Gerson Therapy, inform yourself about it as thoroughly as you can and stay with it. After all, it has the longest and best track record.

Cutting Corners

No one can deny that the Gerson Therapy is labor-intensive; at times, it can feel truly overwhelming. When that happens, patients and/or their caregivers may feel tempted to ease things a little bit by changing the routine (e.g., by preparing all the day's juices in one go and storing them in the refrigerator, instead of making them fresh every hour on the hour as prescribed). This slows the treatment and may lead to failure since **the all-important enzymes in the freshly made juices have a lifespan of some 20 minutes. After that time has elapsed, the minerals, trace elements and most vitamins may survive in the juices, but the living enzymes and their healing power will have been lost.**

Another temptation occurs when some ingredient of the Gerson program becomes hard to obtain, and the patient decides that something else will do just as well in the short term. Extreme caution is needed in such a situation. For instance, if organic carrots are not available, under no circumstances should nonorganic ones be used for juicing (or eating). Commercially grown carrots are saturated with agrochemicals; scrubbing and peeling them will not remove the poisons. As an emergency measure, organic bottled carrot juice may be used on its own or mixed with organic bottled apple juice, **but it should be**

understood that this substitution must only be a short-term solution and not a matter of routine.

One of the worst examples of substitution concerned a woman patient suffering from a collagen disease, who was doing well on the Gerson program until her supply of organic carrots dried up completely. Rather than search for another source, she and her husband decided to substitute orange juice for the elusive carrots, and so she began to drink up to eight glasses of freshly pressed orange juice a day. This would have been harmful to any Gerson patient; in this case, it was disastrous since citrus fruits are counterindicated in all collagen diseases. Her condition deteriorated drastically.

P.S.

Thomas Jefferson wrote, "The price of freedom is eternal vigilance." **Well, the price of getting well is the same: eternal vigilance to avoid pitfalls, resist temptations and decline unasked-for advice from well-meaning outsiders who don't understand what you are doing.** However, you know what you are doing and why, and that is all that matters.

CHAPTER 17 REFERENCE

1.   Anna E. O. Fisher and Declan P. Naughton, "Iron supplements: the quick fix with long-term consequences," *Nutrition Journal* 3 (2) (Jan. 16, 2004).

CHAPTER 18

Taking the New Lifestyle Seriously

Study nature; its eternal laws will keep you.

—*Max Gerson*

The Gerson Therapy is very different from the so-called "normal lifestyle." This makes it difficult for many people to understand its limitations. However, once they understand the reasons for the rules, it is easier to follow them and not cheat.

If and when the cheating becomes too severe, there will be no healing! If the cheating is only "slight," the healing will be slowed down! Depending on the severity of the patient's condition, it is up to each individual to make this choice: **Adhere to the rules to recover, or do not adhere to the rules and interfere with healing.**

Here are some important things to bear in mind:

- The Gerson Therapy is admittedly work intensive. It is almost impossible for a relatively seriously ill patient to work and do the therapy at home for him- or herself.

- **Get help—if only for a few hours in the morning**—to clean the carrots, apples and greens; to make the soup; to prepare the enema concentrate; and to make some of the juices and clean up the machine.

- *Most important:* **Get help to do the housework!** It should not interfere with the preparation of foods and juices. Even if the patient has improved, feels better and looks well, they cannot be expected to take up their "normal" household work, which may include preparing food, doing laundry, dishes, etc., for the rest of the family. Also remember that most household cleansers are toxic. (See Chapter 8, "The Gerson Household," then "Cleaning Chemicals," p. 85.)

- Aside from a rest period of about one hour after lunch, Dr. Gerson felt strongly that the sleep before midnight is the most important sleep. **Don't let television or other items distract you.** If you can't sleep, listen to soft music (without light) and meditate or otherwise relax.

You will also be bombarded with television, radio and newspaper ads, raving about some new treatment or wonder drug. Drugs—whether doctor prescribed, over the counter, or on the street—are invariably liver toxic. Don't trust the hype. Stay with the things of nature!

CHAPTER 19

Frequently Asked Questions

T he Gerson Therapy is so fundamentally different from the usual pill-popping, symptom-centered approach of orthodox medicine that newcomers to this method of healing find some of its details puzzling. It is important to explain the reasons behind the rules; once understood, they prove to be eminently logical. Here is a random selection of the most frequently asked questions with the appropriate answers.

Q: *Why not steam vegetables for a short while, then use the water at the bottom of the pan in the soup, rather than cook all the life out of the vegetables over a long time?*

A: Dr. Gerson was very specific about using the lowest possible heat for cooking vegetables. High heat—steam is hotter than boiling water—changes the colloidal structure of the nutrients, particularly the proteins but also the minerals, and makes them hard to absorb and assimilate. Dr. Gerson even suggested putting a heat disperser under the pan to keep the heat just high enough to simmer the food slowly until well done.

This method does not "cook the life out of the food." The only nutrients that are damaged are the enzymes, which die in temperatures above 140° F (60° C), but patients get a huge supply of enzymes in the fresh raw juices to make up for that loss. The lower heat preserves protein and mineral structures and some vitamins.

Suggesting that the water remaining in the pan should be used acknowledges that the good nutrients, especially the minerals, have been leached out into the water, leaving the cooked vegetables without nutrients! This explains why steamed vegetables have very little taste. Another reason for cooking food slowly at the lowest possible heat is to provide the patient's intestinal tract with "soft bulk" (well-done fiber) to cushion all the raw foods and juices the patient has to consume.

Q: *What about using a B-complex supplement to keep the B vitamins in balance since we use fairly large amounts of B_3 and B_{12}?*

A: Dr. Gerson states in his book[1] that patients were damaged when he administered vitamins B_1 and B_6 to them. The Gerson protocol, with its huge number of juices and fresh foods, is very well balanced and has no need for supplements.

Q: *When can organic soy products be introduced into the diet?*

A: The short answer is ***never***. Soy products of all kinds (e.g., tofu, flour or sauce) contain a substance that blocks absorption of nutrients, besides having a high fat content. **A great deal of research has proven the toxicity of soy, even when grown organically.** The hype claiming soy's usefulness in preventing breast cancer has turned out to be unsubstantiated and the opposite of truth: soy is likely to stimulate malignancy.[2]

Q: *Proper food combining, not mixing starch and fruit, is supposed to be healthy. Why isn't it used on the therapy?*

A: Food combining is probably useful if applied to the average American diet, which is high in animal proteins and sodium (salt). Since all Gerson foods are vegetarian and all vegetables contain a certain amount of starch, it is neither necessary nor possible to separate those two substances.

Q: *Why not supplement vitamins C and E, which help to boost the immune system? Surely one glass of orange juice a day isn't enough?*

A: It is a general misconception that only orange juice contains vitamin C. This is not so. The juices used in the Gerson program are richer in vitamin C than orange juice, and patients consume them in huge quantities every day. Raw salads and fruit increase the intake even further. **Dr. Gerson insisted that no additional vitamins should be given to patients.** Besides, we have found that pharmaceutically produced synthetic vitamins and minerals are poorly absorbed and can even be harmful.

Q: *Potatoes and tomatoes both belong to the deadly nightshade family and are banned from many dietary regimes. Why are they the most used foods on the therapy?*

A: They are not! The most used items are carrots, apples and greens for juicing. Potatoes are extremely nutritious, high in potassium as well as in protein and easily digestible (much more so than rice). Tomatoes are also valuable as they contain vitamins and minerals, including lycopene—a powerful antioxidant that has been extensively researched in recent years and is reputed to boost immune competence.[3] Other vegetables belonging to the nightshade family, such as green peppers and eggplants, are also used in the diet and have never shown any toxic effects.

Q: *How many flare-ups or healing reactions can a patient normally expect?*

A: There is no "normal" number for these. The body produces them as long as it needs to heal. As a rule, the first healing reaction sets in some six to eight days after starting the intensive treatment; the second one comes usually after about six weeks; the third, which is often the most severe, is generally observed after three to three and one-half months. These timings are not fixed and only suggest that the patient can expect healing reactions at certain intervals, which can vary widely in individual cases.

Q: *Are headaches a good sign?*

A: Certainly not. They may be a symptom of flare-ups, when the body is releasing its overload of toxins. In that case, an additional coffee enema should be taken to speed up the process of detoxification. In some rare cases, the toxicity is so high that an enema does not relieve the headache and one or more additional enemas are needed. In almost all patients, as healing progresses, headaches disappear forever, even if they had been a problem for many years. If headaches recur after the therapy has ended, the chances are that exposure to toxins or unsuitable food has occurred and must be avoided in the future.

Q: *When do patients begin to feel better and have more energy?*

A: Almost all patients, including extremely ill ones, feel better after the first week on the therapy. Pain diminishes, appetite returns and sleep improves. All this adds up to a great psychological boost. It also signals the moment when the patient has to be warned about an impending healing reaction, bringing with it days of feeling unwell. A true rise in energy may occur in three to six months, depending on the age and condition of the patient. At that point, it is most important that the patient continues to rest and doesn't launch into multiple activities! The new energy must be used for healing and nothing else. There will be plenty of time later to build muscles and make up for lost exercise time. Trying to do so too soon can result in a serious setback.

Q: *Are there any circumstances under which a Gerson patient should use antibiotics?*

A: Yes, but such circumstances are rare. Since virtually all medical drugs have a toxic component, **Gerson patients are advised not to take any prescription or nonprescription items.** Antibiotics are the exception. While in general medical practice they have been seriously over-used, weakening the immune system[4] and producing resistant bacteria,[5] very occasionally they need to be used by patients whose immune system is seriously weakened.

Since it may take considerable time to restore the patient's immune system, in a case of acute infection, antibiotics are required. We use them to help fight colds and attacks of flu, and patients undergoing dental work should take them as recommended by their dentist. **Of course, antibiotics don't kill viruses, but they can control the opportunistic infections that attack a weakened body.** For colds, we use the least toxic antibiotics, namely penicillin, unless the patient is allergic to it. For other infections, the appropriate antibiotic has to be chosen. For patients on the Gerson Therapy, adding one aspirin, one 500 mg tablet of vitamin C, and 50 mg of niacin, taken together with the antibiotic, greatly increases the effectiveness of the latter without the need to increase the dosage.

Q: *Carrot juice is high in sugars. Does that not disturb the healing of diabetes?*

A: No. Carrot juice forms a very important part of healing. Rather than disturbing recovery, carrot juice provides the best source of vitamin A as well as most other vitamins. It is also one of the most complete sources of minerals containing most of the essential minerals in easily absorbed form. It is even high in vegetarian proteins and, for those reasons, it is an excellent source of total nutrition and healing.

Q: *With all the enemas being used in the course of the two years on the therapy, will I become dependent on enemas forever?*

A: No. Many patients, particularly women, have been constipated for some time, often for many years. When the liver and intestines are fully restored, most patients become "regular" again. Many of those who had been constipated recover "regularity." If not, it would be foolish to jeopardize recovery, when enemas are so important to heal and restore the body, just to be sure to remain "regular." In case the patient does lose their regularity, at worst they will have to take a daily enema as a morning routine. Dr. Gerson emphatically stressed, "Never let the sun set on a day when you haven't moved your bowel!"

Q: *On this therapy, without animal products, where do I get my proteins?*

A: As we have seen above, most vegetables contain adequate amounts of protein. This type of nutrient is easily absorbed, well digested and assimilated so that it produces healing—rather than feeding—tumor tissue, causing arthritic conditions, damaging kidneys, etc. The strongest and largest land animals (e.g., elephants, bulls and orangutans) are vegetarians and obtain their proteins from grass, plants, leaves and fruit. Carrot juice is high in proteins as are potatoes, oatmeal and most vegetables.

CHAPTER 19 REFERENCES

1. M. Gerson, *A Cancer Therapy: Results of Fifty Cases and The Cure of Advanced Cancer by Diet Therapy: A Summary of Thirty Years of Clinical Experimentation,* 6th ed. (San Diego, CA: Gerson Institute, 1999), Appendix II, p. 418.
2. G. Matrone, et al., "Effect of Genistin on Growth and Development of the Male Mouse," *Journal of Nutrition* (1956): 235-240.
3. "Tomatoes, Tomato-Based Products, Lycopene, and Cancer: Review of the Epidemiologic Literature," *Journal of the National Cancer Institute* 91 (4) (Feb. 17, 1999): 317-331.
4. www.natural-cures-ear-sinus-infections.com/Antibiotic-Overuse.html
5. C. Woteki, J. Henney, *Strategy to Address the Problem of Agricultural Antimicrobial Use and the Emergence of Resistance.* FDA. Electronically published 10/2009; originally published 9/14/00 [cited 2010 0602]. Accessible at: www.fda.gov/downloads/animalveterinary/safetyhealth/antimicrobialresistance/UCM134773.pdf.

CHAPTER 20

Life After Gerson

C oming off the therapy at the right time has to be handled with care. Determining the right time is a tricky issue. To stop too soon, before all the essential organs are restored, is a great mistake, likely to lead to a recurrence. Patients suffering from nonmalignant diseases which respond well to the Gerson Therapy can be fully healed in a year or 18 months.

While coming off the treatment too soon is unwise, staying on it for "too long" does no harm. Stopping the therapy has to be a gradual process, slowly reducing the juices—if all goes well—reducing enemas to possibly two a week if the patient now has normal daily bowel movements and pain or headaches (symptoms of toxicity). Juices may be cut down to five or six a day, preferably indefinitely.

Eating Wisely

Changing over from the strict dietary rules to a more permissive regime also needs care. During the treatment, the body has gotten used to the best possible nutrition: fresh, pure, tasty, organic vegetarian food that is easily digested and provides all the necessary nutrients for health and fitness. It would be a grave mistake to switch from such a wholesome diet to the so-called normal variety—heavy with meat, poultry, cheese and chemically rich convenience foods—and risk a serious upset.

In our experience, recovered patients with their "clean" systems don't feel tempted by such foods even if, during the long treatment, they did fantasize about some "forbidden fruit." On the saltless Gerson regime, their taste buds have recovered from the paralysis caused by the highly salty foods of the past; now they find anything salty unpleasant and even offensive. (This is similar to former smokers who find it impossible to stay in a smoky room, let alone start smoking again.)

Of course, once a recovered patient is in a truly good condition with their systems working well, it is all right to attend a banquet, a wedding or a birthday celebration and "binge" a little. Afterwards, digestive enzymes should be taken for a few days, accompanied by a daily enema, to get rid of the mess and feel good again. **Please don't discard your enema bucket.** "Upside-down coffee," in Gerson parlance, helps if you have a headache, a toothache or even an incipient cold or a general malaise. Also, hang on to your Norwalk or other juicer instead of switching over to bottled juices; they won't help keep you well.

Patients who had been very seriously ill must take extra precautions to preserve their newfound health. **We suggest that, however long they have been off the therapy, they should go back on the full intensive program for two weeks, twice a year.** (Spring and fall, the times of seasonal changes, are best for this purpose.) During those two weeks, they should drink 10 to 13 juices a day, eat only freshly prepared organic foods, avoid animal proteins and take three or more enemas daily. If this return to the strict Gerson protocol produces a healing reaction, which these patients would recognize at once, the body is obviously clearing up some fresh damage and the strict program should be extended for another two weeks. If, however, no new symptoms pop up, the patient is doing well and can stop the "refresher course" after two weeks.

The Art of Maintenance

Originally, Dr. Gerson suggested that recovered patients should maintain their good health by ensuring that 75% of their diet con-

sisted of "protective" foods—namely, organic fruits and vegetables high in nutrients, vitamins, minerals and enzymes—to keep the immune system in prime condition. The remaining 25% of food was to be "at choice." Unfortunately, this division is no longer applicable since the freely chosen foods would be far too damaging. We therefore have to urge former patients to stay with 90% of "protective" foods and have at most 10% of their intake consist of freely chosen items.

Even so, they should never return to fast foods, junk foods containing pesticides, food additives and other toxic stuff, and most certainly not items such as hot dogs, spiced meats and sausages laced with preservatives or cheese—the very foods that contributed to the breakdown of their health in the first place. However, if some serious dietary indiscretion occurs, it is wise to go back on the full therapy for a few weeks and clear up the body rather than risk long-term damage. **Obviously, great care must be taken with alcohol; very occasionally, a little wine may be enjoyed, but only if it is organic.** Commercially produced wines, made from frequently sprayed grapes, are to be avoided.

If you know what to avoid and what to hang on to, maintenance quickly becomes an easy and pleasant routine. **The answer to the question, "Is there life after Gerson?," is a clear and resounding yes!**

Overcoming Stress and Tension

The Gerson program will also work best for the relaxed, unstressed patient. After all, it is not enough to eat the best possible food and drink the most health-giving juices; they also have to be digested and absorbed properly. It is no secret that anxiety and worry can wreak havoc with digestion.

Keeping mind and emotions on an even keel, banishing stress and fear must be part of the Gerson patient's daily routine. Fortunately, there are some simple, enjoyable methods that make this possible. In this chapter, we present a full range. Please try them and which suit you best.

Minding the Body

Posture can have a huge impact on how we feel, just as how we feel is often betrayed by our posture. When we are happy, we walk on air. When we are miserable, our head goes down, our shoulders move up and our back curves forward and slumps—all of which compress our innards and add to the gloom. That will never do.

Learn to keep your spine straight but not rigid, both standing and sitting. (Please freeze for a moment and check what your spine is doing.)

Sit with both feet on the ground and don't cross your legs; doing so impedes the circulation and twists the spine. Walk from the hips and avoid leaning forward, as if you were pushing a grocery cart. You can't get ahead of yourself! Think of your head as the hook of a coat hanger, with your body hanging from it loosely and comfortably. The shoulders are a particularly tension-prone part of the body. They tend to move forward and up, whenever we feel stressed, as if wanting to protect the chest. A side effect of this unconscious move is that anxious people seem to have short necks. In the memorable words of a yoga teacher, opening up your chest means saying yes to life.

Make sure your shoulders are where they belong. Stand up straight, draw both shoulders up as far as they will go, right up to the earlobes, and then drop them as if they had become redundant. Where they land is their natural position. Please memorize it for future use.

It is also helpful to keep your neck supple and relaxed (and make it longer!) by regular exercise. Turn your head slowly from left to right and back. Drop your head gently forward and backward, keeping your lower jaw loose. Rotate your head first clockwise, then counterclockwise, repeating each movement five times. If at any time you feel you are tensing up, imagine that you are a rag doll in a strong breeze and move accordingly.

Hands are also tension-prone. They tend to curl into fists as soon as we feel anxious or angry. In old Western films, you could tell that things were getting dangerous when the hero's knuckles turned white. Actually, anybody's knuckles can turn white from fear and this is what needs to be avoided. Train yourself to keep your fingers splayed when your hands are at rest. That prevents the tensing up of the arms, which would lead to further tension rushing through the body. If at first you fail and all you have are fists, imagine that you have washed your hands and have no towel, so that you need to shake both hands vigorously from the wrists. As you do that, feel the tension dropping away from your fingertips.

Breathing deserves our full attention. Breath is the basic condition of life. We can live for quite a while without food and for a much shorter time without water, but life without breath ends in a few moments.

Most of us neglect this vital function until we learn otherwise and switch from shallow to deep abdominal breathing. This way, routinely used by singers, speakers, practitioners of yoga and athletes, boosts the body's oxygen intake and has a calming effect.

The method is simplicity itself. With each in-breath, push out your stomach so that the breath can fill your lungs to full capacity. Fill your lower lungs first, then the middle of your lungs and finally your upper lungs. Hold your breath for a second or two and then, as you breathe out, pull in your stomach hard, squeezing out the stale air. Find your own rhythm and practice this method several times a day until it becomes your natural way of breathing. If at first it is a bit difficult, imagine that, in your abdomen, there is a beautiful balloon, which you inflate with each in-breath and deflate by letting the air out. You will be surprised what a difference better breathing makes to your well-being.

Matters of the Mind

Your mental attitude can be your best ally—or your worst enemy— and the same applies to your imagination, depending on how you use it. Positively used, your thoughts and ideas can help you to reprogram your entire outlook, your moods and your feelings so that they promote health and healing instead of dragging you down. Energy follows thought!

There are several ways to achieve the best possible state of mind. All of them depend on your ability to relax as fully as possible so that no tension interferes with what you are trying to do. The simplest way is to lie on your back on a comfortable but not too soft surface, with your hands loosely resting by your sides. Close your eyes. Start breathing slowly, deeply, from the abdomen. With each in-breath, imagine drawing in brilliant light, which fills you with peace, strength and energy. With each out-breath, imagine releasing all tiredness, tension, pain or anxiety in the shape of dirty, dark smoke. Let your head and your body become very heavy so that the floor carries your weight. Check through your body, starting with your toes and working your way up to the top of your head, for traces of tension or stiffness, and release them.

Make sure your jaw is relaxed and your tongue lies easy against your upper palate. Stay with this feeling of peace, release and relaxation for a little while.

This basic letting-go is the key to all kinds of inner work, including meditation, prayer, visualization and affirmations. Practiced at least twice a day, free from disturbance, noise and interruptions, it will make a great difference to your mental state, which in turn will affect your body.

Meditation

Meditation is a simple way to still the ever-busy brain and enter a place of profound stillness and peace which, for a short while, lets us escape from everyday reality. It needs practice; the brain is hard to discipline and keeps bringing in thoughts, fragments of ideas and all kinds of mental rubbish. At first, you may find that even 30 seconds of stillness is quite an achievement. Don't give up! There are ways to improve the situation.

One way is to get hold of intruding thoughts, identify them, imagine tying a big balloon to each one and watch them float away. Another way is to improve concentration by counting from one to four, seeing in your mind's eye the numbers, shining bright and beautiful against a dark curtain, and repeat the counting 10 times. You can also place a clock at eye level and fix your entire attention to the second hand going round and round so that nothing else matters. Gradually—but with perseverance—you'll find it easier to achieve spells of thought-free awareness, leading to an extraordinary sense of restfulness and peace.

Switching off the brain for a little while also enables us to hear our so-called inner voice—the voice of intuition and wisdom. Whatever our belief system, and whether or not we are religious, we all have an inner life and a set of values by which we live. Often, it is at a time of crisis, caused by a serious health breakdown, that we turn inward and review our position in life. Naturally, Gerson patients are totally free to choose their own way in this field; we are all different and must respect our differences. However, it is the experience of many doctors, counselors and other health professionals that patients who believe in a higher reality, who are able to pray and put their faith in God, fare better than those who don't. Prayer, coming from the heart, with trust in the ultimate rightness of things, can be a great support on the rocky path of recovery.

Visualization

Visualization uses the imagination to reprogram not only the mind but, to a certain extent, the body. It works through images, bypassing the thinking-talking brain, and those images come from the same deep area of the psyche as the ones we meet in our dreams. The purpose of visualization is to prescribe, so to speak, what we want to achieve: defeating disease, rebuilding health, recovering and living a full life. Using visualization in the context of cancer was first developed in the 1970s by the American radiation oncologist Carl Simonton, MD. *Getting Well Again,*[1] the book he wrote with his then-wife, psychologist Stephanie Matthews-Simonton, has appeared in many editions and several languages.

The essence of the Simonton technique is to find one image for the disease and another one for the treatment, and how the latter attacks and gradually demolishes the former. For instance, in the state of deep relaxation described above, the Gerson patient may visualize his or her tumor as a big blob of black mud, and the juices as powerful bursts of golden liquid that attack and gradually clear away the mud. Read cold from the page, this may sound odd; practiced as it is meant to be, it can be a powerful experience.

Here is a simple visualization exercise for daily use: yourself in a perfectly beautiful place, real or imaginary, where you feel safe, secure and happy. Make yourself comfortable in imagination, in whatever way feels right for you: gently swaying in a soft hammock, walking in a perfect garden or sitting happily with a loved one. Choose your own setting outside time and space and be refreshed by its peace and beauty.

Now yourself as you wish to be: healthy, fit, strong and active, doing the things you most enjoy, able to give and receive love and feeling at home in the world. Surrender to this image, become it and anchor it in your mind and heart, then slowly return to mundane reality but bring with you the memory of the experience. It does make a difference. Actually, a similar technique is used by successful sportsmen and sportswomen who, before an important event, visualize themselves doing extremely well in their chosen area.

Imagination is powerful. Used well, it stimulates and tunes the body. It is free, nontoxic and has no harmful side effects, which makes it the ideal supplementary tool for Gerson patients.

CHAPTER 21 REFERENCE

1. Carl Simonton, MD, James L. Creighton and Stephanie Matthews-Simonton, *Getting Well Again* (New York: Bantam Books, reissue edition April 1, 1992).

CHAPTER 22

Recipes

L ast, but far from least, this chapter contains a treasury of recipes that add variety, pleasure and super-healthy nutrition to Gerson-style meals. However, there are some important points to remember:

- Study and learn by heart the basic rules for food preparation described in Chapter 11, "Preparing Food and Juices—The Basic Rules," p. 103.

- If you are a Gerson patient, newly embarked on the full therapy, you need to limit your food intake to the basic recipes contained in that chapter for the first three months and eat no dairy products for the first six to 10 weeks.

- After three months, you may introduce some variety by using different salads, dressings and vegetable courses.

- The "Special Soup or Hippocrates Soup" and the baked potato are essential parts of the healing diet and must not be omitted.

If you are not ill but wish to improve your health and well-being by switching to the Gerson lifestyle, you may of course enjoy the recipes freely. Please use the slow, low heat, waterless or minimum-water cooking method, described in Chapter 12, in order to preserve precious nutrients.

Patients diagnosed with collagen diseases should avoid citrus fruit and orange or grapefruit juices. Use freshly pressed apple juice or apple/carrot juice in their place.

Special Notes

Bread

You will find no recipes for bread or other flour-based baked goods in this chapter. The only acceptable bread—unsalted, organic 100% rye bread—is available at good health food stores, so there is no point in baking bread at home. Patients are allowed two small slices of bread a day, but only after eating the complete Gerson meals consisting of salad, soup and potato with vegetables and fruit. Bread must not take the place of any of these items.

Yogurt

Yogurt, when permitted, must be certified organic and fat free (or extremely low fat). A few recipes refer to "yogurt." To make this, hang some regular yogurt, placed in several layers of cheesecloth, over the sink or in a cheesecloth-lined strainer over a bowl, and allow it to drain overnight

Sweeteners

The only permitted sweeteners are:

- Organic raw brown sugar, which is available in various shades ranging from light beige to dark brown

- Organic clear honey

- Organic maple syrup

- Unsulphured molasses

- Sucanat (also known as rapadura)

In the recipes, these ingredients are referred to as "honey" and "sugar."

Washing Fruits and Vegetables

All fruits and vegetables must be washed before use. If the water supply in your area is not fluoridated, purified water (produced by reverse osmosis) may be used, both for washing produce and for cooking. If the water supply contains fluoride, only distilled water is permissible for cooking and as a final rinse for fruits and vegetables. (For distillers, see Chapter 8, "The Gerson Household," p. 79.)

Baking

When baking, the oven should always be preheated.

Cooking Time/Serving Size

When a specific cooking time or a number of people served is omitted, it is because it depends on the size of the ingredients. For example, if a large potato is used, it takes much more time to bake or cook than a small one. Also, one or two large potatoes serve more people than the same number of small ones.

Special Soup or Hippocrates Soup

"Special Soup" or "Hippocrates Soup" are interchangeable terms for the same staple item of the Gerson diet. In some recipes, it is referred to as "soup stock." For a detailed description, see Chapter 11, "Preparing Food and Juices—The Basic Rules," p. 103.

Bon appetit!

Recipes

Dips

Carrot and Dill Dip

Preparation time: 15 minutes
Cooking time: 30 minutes
Serves 4-8

1 lb. carrots, scrubbed, unpeeled
4 tbsp. yogurt
2 tbsp. dill weed (or 2 tsp. dried dill), finely chopped
1 tsp. flaxseed oil
juice of 1 small lemon

Simmer carrots until just tender. Drain and leave until cooled. Put through the food mill. Mix in yogurt, dill, flaxseed oil and lemon juice. Mix well. Chill in the refrigerator. Serve as part of a large salad or as a dip with carrot, zucchini and bell pepper sticks. Also delicious on bread.

Orange (or Red) Pepper Dip

Preparation time: 15 minutes
Serves 6

2 orange (or red) bell peppers

10 oz. yogurt

1/2 tsp. organic tomato purée

Seed and dice one of the peppers very finely and mix with the yogurt and tomato purée. Slice the remaining pepper lengthwise in half and remove the seeds. Place the yogurt mixture into each pepper half. Place on a serving dish with thin strips of carrot, zucchini and celery.

Appetizers

Celery Root Rémoulade Appetizer

Preparation Time: 10 minutes
Serves 2-4

celery root
radicchio lettuce
2 or 3 varieties of loose leaf lettuce (butter or red leaf lettuce)
green onions (or chives), chopped
parsley (or tarragon)

Dressing:
vinegar
water
honey
yogurt

Combine the dressing ingredients. Grate the celery root and add the dressing. Place lettuce leaves on a plate and top with celery root. Sprinkle with chopped green onions (or chives) and parsley (or tarragon).

Eggplant Appetizer

Preparation time: 15 minutes
Cooking time: 50 minutes
Serves 2

1 eggplant
1 small onion, chopped
1/2 tbsp. organic tomato purée
parsley (or cilantro)
lemon wedge
yogurt

Prick the skin of the eggplant all over. Place directly onto the oven rack (or use a small baking dish) and bake at 375° F (190° C) for about 40 minutes near the top of the oven, turning once after 20 minutes.

Remove from oven and cool. When cool, peel away the stalk and skin, and chop the flesh until you have a rough purée. Heat a little water in a small pan and sauté the chopped onion over low heat for about 10 minutes or until soft. Stir in the tomato purée and the eggplant purée. Cook for another 2 minutes over high heat to remove excess moisture. Remove from heat and cool completely. Chop some parsley (or cilantro) and mix in with the purée. Lay on a bed of lettuce. Garnish with a wedge of lemon and a little yogurt.

Grapefruit Appetizer

Preparation time: 15 minutes
Serves 1 or 2

1 pink grapefruit
celery
1 red bell pepper, seeded
radicchio (or red leaf lettuce leaves)
grated horseradish

Cut the grapefruit in half. Juice one-half and cut out the segments of the other half. Chop some celery and seeded red pepper. Arrange a layer of radicchio (or red leaf lettuce leaves) on a plate. Mix grapefruit segments, celery and red pepper together and put on top of lettuce. Make a dressing with grapefruit juice flavored with a little grated horseradish (or chopped mint leaves).

Variation: Put grapefruit segments on top of endive and watercress. Make a dressing with yogurt and a little grapefruit juice. Mix well and serve immediately.

How to segment a grapefruit: Cut a horizontal slice off the top and bottom. Sit the grapefruit flat and, using a sharp knife, remove the peel and outer white membrane by cutting downwards in sections. Using a container to catch any juice, cut between the membranes and the flesh of each segment to the core, taking care to point the knife blade away from you. Work around the grapefruit, easing out each segment as you go.

Jerusalem Artichoke Paté

Preparation time: 20 minutes
Cooking time: 40 minutes
Serves 2

1 lb. Jerusalem artichokes
1 tbsp. yogurt
1-2 tsp. lemon juice
parsley, chopped
flaxseed oil

Scrub the artichokes. Put in dish in oven to roast at 400° F (204° C) for
25 minutes. (It's a good idea to cook them with your baked potato.)
Allow to cool and remove skin. Mash or purée (with electric blender or
food mill) until it has a creamy consistency. Add the yogurt, lemon
juice, chopped parsley and flaxseed oil, and beat together. Serve as an
appetizer or a snack with toasted slices of bread and a smattering of various lettuce leaves and cherry tomatoes to decorate.

Melon and Mango Appetizer

Preparation time: 15 minutes
Serves 2-4

slices of honeydew and/or cantaloupe melon
slices of mango

Dressing:
1/2 tbsp. honey
1 tbsp. flaxseed oil
2 tbsp. lime (or lemon) juice
mint leaves

Cut the melon in half and remove the rind. Slice the melon and arrange
in a fan shape on a shallow plate. Slice the mango lengthwise and peel,
including the flesh left around the pit. Cut the mango flesh into slices
and arrange between the melon slices on the plate. Pour the dressing
over the melon.

Papaya and Lime Appetizer

Preparation time: 15 minutes
Serves 2

2 papayas
2 tbsp. honey
juice of 1 lime
1 lime for decoration, sliced

Peel the papaya and remove the seeds. Cut into slices (or cubes). Mix the honey with the lime juice and pour over papaya slices. Toss gently and refrigerate. Serve chilled, decorated with thin slices of lime.

Stuffed Zucchini Appetizer

Preparation time: 10 minutes
Cooking time: 5 minutes
Serves 2-4

8 medium zucchinis
1 large onion, chopped
1 green bell pepper
3 tomatoes
1 tsp. parsley, chopped
1 clove garlic, crushed
red leaf lettuce
4-6 tbsp. dressing

Dressing:
6 tbsp. apple cider vinegar (or lemon juice)
4 tbsp. water
herbs
flaxseed oil

Cook the zucchini whole (about 5 minutes on a very low heat) until half-cooked. Cut off both ends and cut each in half lengthwise. Scoop out the seeds and chop them. Sprinkle some dressing into the zucchini hollows and add a little chopped onion. Leave to marinate while preparing the stuffing. Take the remaining onion and chop the pepper and tomatoes, add the chopped parsley and crushed garlic, and mix with the chopped zucchini middles. Toss in the rest of the dressing and fill the hollows with the mixture. Arrange on a layer of red leaf lettuce to serve.

Yogurt and Apricot Sorbet Appetizer

Freezing time: 2-3 hours
Preparation time: 15 minutes
Cooking time: 40 minutes
Serves 2-4

8 oz. dried apricots
20 fl. oz. water
10 oz. yogurt
2 tbsp. honey

Place the apricots and a little water in a saucepan and bring to a boil. Cover and simmer for 30-40 minutes, or until soft. Add the rest of the water to bring the liquid content to 15 oz. Leave to cool. Place the apricots and liquid in a blender and blend until smooth. Add the yogurt and honey but do not blend these. Transfer the contents to a freeze-proof container and freeze until solid. Use an ice-cream scooper to serve one or two scoops into a bowl. Serve immediately.

Dressings

Baba Ghanoush (Eggplant and Lemon Dressing)

Preparation time: 10 minutes
Cooking time: 1 hour
Serves 3 or 4

1 large eggplant
1 or 2 cloves garlic
2 tbsp. lemon juice
1 tbsp. parsley, chopped

Bake the eggplant for 1 hour at 350-400° F (177-204° C). When cooled enough to peel, drain off excess juice, squeezing gently. Mash and blend with garlic until fairly smooth and add lemon juice and parsley. Mix well. Serve with lemon wedges. Good with crudités (raw veggies) and as a relish as well as a sauce.

Variation: Mix with yogurt.

Basic Salad Dressing

Preparation time: 7 minutes
Serves 2

2 tbsp. lemon juice (or apple cider vinegar)
2 tbsp. water
pinch of sugar (optional)

Mix together and put into a container with any of the following:
tarragon, pushed in stalk first
shallots (or green onions), finely chopped
2 cloves garlic, peeled and crushed
fresh bay leaf
lemon grass (for a lemon flavor)

Dressing for Vegetables

Preparation time: 5 minutes
Serves 2

2 tbsp. lemon juice (or apple cider vinegar)
2 tbsp. water
pinch of sugar (optional)
yogurt

Mix lemon juice (or apple cider vinegar), water and sugar (if used). Mix in yogurt and beat well.

Flaxseed Oil and Lemon Juice Dressing

Preparation time: 5 minutes
Serves 2

1 tbsp. flaxseed oil
1/2 tbsp. lemon juice
(Use a ratio of 2/3 oil to 1/3 lemon juice)
garlic
fresh herbs
a little orange juice

Combine all the ingredients in a pitcher and stir vigorously. Pour over the salad and serve immediately.

Garlic and Green Onion Dressing

Preparation time: 5 minutes
Serves 1

1 tbsp. flaxseed oil
1/2 tbsp. lemon juice (or apple cider vinegar)
1 clove garlic
1 green onion
fresh parsley
chives
dill
fennel
a little mint

Mix flaxseed oil with lemon juice (or apple cider vinegar). Crush the garlic and add. Chop the green onion, parsley and chives and add, together with the dill, fennel and mint. Either pour over the salad and serve immediately, or put into a pitcher and allow guests to serve themselves.

Variation: If you have no fresh herbs, use a generous pinch of suitable dried herbs.

Basic Dressing

Preparation time: 5 minutes
Serves 6

2-1/3 cup apple cider vinegar
1 tsp. sugar
2/3 cup water

Mix ingredients together.

Variation: Add some or all of the following herbs (optional), letting them infuse: tarragon (pushed in stalk first); shallots or spring onions, finely chopped; 2 cloves of garlic, peeled and crushed with the back of a knife; and 1 fresh bay leaf.

Orange Vinaigrette

Preparation time: 6 minutes
Serves 1

1 clove garlic
2 tbsp. fresh parsley
2 tbsp. apple cider vinegar
1 tsp. sugar
4 tbsp. orange juice
1 tbsp. flaxseed oil

Chop the garlic and parsley, and add to vinegar, sugar, orange juice and flaxseed oil.

Yogurt, Garlic and Honey Dressing

Preparation time: 6 minutes
Serves 2

6 oz. yogurt
1 clove garlic, crushed
1 tsp. honey
watercress

Mix the ingredients, toss lightly and serve immediately. Garnish with watercress.

Yogurt, Herb and Vinegar Dressing

Preparation time: 4 minutes

apple cider vinegar
a little water
honey
yogurt
parsley
tarragon

Mix all together.

Yogurt, Onion and Apple Cider Vinegar Dressing

Preparation time: 4 minutes

yogurt
apple cider vinegar
chopped onion

Mix all together and serve with a green salad.

Salads

Apple and Carrot Salad

Preparation time: 15 minutes
Serves 2

1 small crisp red apple
1 large carrot
1 green onion, chopped
1 radish, sliced
apple juice
mint

Grate the apple and carrot into a dish and add a chopped green onion and a sliced radish. Pour over a little apple juice and sprinkle with mint. Serve on a bed of mixed colored salad leaves, such as radicchio, watercress or parsley.

Beet and Watercress Salad

Preparation time: 5 minutes

cooked beet
flaxseed oil
watercress

Chop cooked beet and toss in a little flaxseed oil. Serve with watercress.

Beet Salad Yolande

Preparation time: 20 minutes

cooked beets
carrots
celery
apples
parsley

Dressing:
yogurt
lemon juice
flaxseed oil

Dice the beets, carrots, celery and apples and put into a bowl. Make the dressing and mix in with the vegetables. Sprinkle with parsley.

Beet Thermidor

Preparation time: 6 minutes

cooked beets

Dressing:
yogurt

lemon juice
grated horseradish

Dice cooked beets, put into a bowl and add the dressing.

Carrot Salad

Preparation time: 15 minutes
Serves 2-4

8 oz. carrots
1 medium crisp eating apple
5 oz. yogurt
juice of 1 large orange

Grate the carrots into a bowl. Cut the apple into quarters, remove core, then grate into the bowl and mix with the carrot. Mix the yogurt with the orange juice and stir into the salad.

Variation: Presoaked raisins (soak overnight in cold water, or pour boiling water over them and leave for a couple of hours until plump) or sultanas can also be added.

Carrot and Orange Salad with Fresh Dates

Preparation time: 15 minutes
Serves 2

1 large carrot
1 orange
a few fresh dates
toasted oats

Dressing:
lemon (or lime) juice
flaxseed oil

Cut the carrot into thin strips. Segment the orange and mix with the carrot. Chop the dates and add. Add dressing and garnish with toasted oats.

Carrot and Raisin Salad

Preparation time: 10 minutes*
* Does not include presoaking
Serves 2

3 large carrots, grated
2 oz. raisins, presoaked
lettuce
2 tsp. parsley, chopped

Dressing:
1 clove garlic, crushed
flaxseed oil
apple cider vinegar
1/2 tsp. honey
2 tsp. lemon juice

Mix grated raw carrots with presoaked raisins (soak the raisins overnight in cold water, or pour boiling water over them and leave for a couple of hours until plump). Add dressing and serve on lettuce garnished with chopped parsley.

Carrot, Apple and Onion Salad

Preparation time: 15 minutes
Serves 2

12 oz. carrots
8 oz. apples
1 medium onion
10 oz. yogurt
juice of 1/2 lemon

Shred the carrots, apples and onion. Combine with the yogurt and lemon juice. Serve with a mixed green salad.

Celery Salad

Preparation time: 10 minutes
Serves 2

2 stalks celery
2 crisp small eating apples
1/4 medium red bell pepper, finely sliced
mixed lettuce leaves

Dressing:
apple cider vinegar
flaxseed oil
1 tsp. honey

Chop the celery and apples and put into a large bowl. Add the finely sliced red bell pepper. Add the dressing. Line a salad plate with mixed lettuce leaves and pile the dressed salad on top.

Cherry Tomato and Watercress Relish

Preparation time: 15 minutes
Serves 2-4

cherry tomatoes (red and yellow)
watercress
fresh chives (or green onions), finely chopped
herbs, finely chopped

Halve the tomatoes and place in a bowl. Steam the watercress over boiling water for 10 seconds, rinse well in cold water and shake dry. Trim off any woody stems and cut or tear the remaining stems and leaves into small pieces. Add to the tomatoes. Add the finely chopped chives (or green onions) and herbs and toss together.

Chicory and Orange Salad

Preparation time: 15 minutes
Serves 2-4

1 lb. chicory heads

2 large oranges
1 medium green onion
juice of 1/2 lemon
1 tbsp. flaxseed oil
1 tsp. honey

Trim the chicory and slice into rounds about 1/2-inch thick. Push the rounds apart to make rings. Peel the oranges, removing the white pith, and slice into rounds. Place the chicory in a bowl and lay the oranges in overlapping rings around the top, leaving the center empty. Trim and chop the green onion and sprinkle into the center. Mix the lemon juice, flaxseed oil and honey, and pour over the salad. Leave for a few minutes before serving to allow the flavors to "marry."

Coleslaw

*Preparation time: 15 minutes**
* Does not include presoaking

raisins
white cabbage
apple
celery
onion

Dressing:
yogurt
lemon juice
flaxseed oil

Presoak the raisins (soak the raisins overnight in cold water, or pour boiling water over them and leave for a couple of hours until plump). Thinly shred the white cabbage and apple. Finely chop the celery and onion. Put all into a bowl and add the raisins. Toss in dressing.

Colorful Mixed Salad

Preparation time: 15 minutes
Serves 2

zucchini
beet
apple
lettuce
tomato
orange

Dressing:
equal amounts of apple cider vinegar and water
honey (or maple syrup)
garlic
lemon (or orange) juice

Grate the zucchini, beet and apple. Add the dressing and mix them together or pile them in separate mounds onto a bed of lettuce. Decorate with slices of tomatoes and orange.

Colorful Three-Cabbage Salad

Preparation time: 15 minutes*
* Does not include presoaking
Serves 2

2 oz. raisins
4 oz. each white, red and green cabbage
4 oz. carrot
1 medium onion, finely sliced
1 small crisp eating apple, chopped
watercress

Dressing:
5 fl. oz. yogurt
a little flaxseed oil
1 clove garlic, crushed

Presoak the raisins (soak the raisins overnight in cold water, or pour boiling water over them and leave for a couple of hours until plump). Finely shred the cabbage. Grate the carrot. Put both in a bowl with the raisins, finely sliced onion and chopped apple. Mix well. Mix the dressing ingredients and pour over the salad just before serving, tossing lightly. Garnish with watercress.

Colorful Winter Salad

Preparation time: 20 minutes
Serves 4-6

3 tart eating apples
lemon juice
1/4 medium-sized red cabbage
1 medium carrot
1/2 medium red bell pepper
2 sticks celery
1/2 red onion
watercress

Core and roughly chop the apples and mix with lemon juice in a small bowl. Core and finely shred the red cabbage. Peel and grate the carrot. (This is the only time to peel the carrots. If they are grated with their skins on, they tend to turn brown.) Seed and chop the red pepper. Slice the celery. Peel and chop the red onion. Put all the above ingredients into a large bowl. Garnish with watercress.

Variations: Serve with cottage cheese (unsalted and uncreamed or fat-free) and your favorite dressing.

Crunchy Salad

Preparation time: 15 minutes*
* Does not include presoaking
Serves 4-6

2 oz. dried apricots, chopped
3 oz. raisins

1 lb. white cabbage
1 green bell pepper
1 red bell pepper (or 1/2 bunch of radishes)
watercress

Dressing:
6 fl. oz. yogurt
1 clove garlic, crushed
1 tsp. honey

Presoak the apricots and raisins (soak overnight in cold water, or pour boiling water over them and leave for a couple of hours until plump). Finely shred the white cabbage. Chop the pepper (or radishes). Place into a bowl together with the raisins and chopped apricots. Mix well. Mix the dressing and pour over the salad. Toss lightly, garnish with watercress and serve.

Endive and Orange Salad

Preparation time: 15 minutes
Serves 2

1 small head of endive
1 red bell pepper
2 oranges
2 tomatoes
1 tbsp. herbs, chopped

Dressing:
juice of 2 oranges
5 oz. yogurt
1 tsp. honey

Chop the endive and put into a bowl. Seed the pepper, cut into thin strips and add to the bowl. Peel the oranges, removing the pith with the peel. Cut out segments between the membranes and add to the bowl with the tomatoes. Make the dressing and toss into the salad. Sprinkle with chopped herbs.

Fruity Winter Salad

Preparation time: 15 minutes*
* Does not include presoaking
Serves 2-4

2 oz. raisins
2 oz. dried figs
2 oz. dried apricots
1/2 white cabbage
2 carrots
2 red eating apples
8 tbsp. yogurt
1 lemon
parsley, chopped

Presoak the raisins, figs and apricots (soak overnight in cold water, or pour boiling water over them and leave for a couple of hours until plump). Finely shred the cabbage. Coarsely grate the carrots and apples. (Sprinkle the apples with lemon juice to stop them from turning brown.) Put the above ingredients into a bowl. Combine the yogurt, lemon juice and chopped parsley in a jug and spoon over the salad. Toss together until well mixed.

Gerson Coleslaw

Preparation time: 15 minutes
Serves 2-4

onion
white cabbage
carrot

Dressing:
2 tbsp. lemon juice
2 tbsp. water
sugar (optional)
yogurt
cottage cheese (unsalted and uncreamed or fat-free)

Slice or chop the onion. Grate or slice the white cabbage. Grate the carrot. Mix all together. For the dressing, mix lemon juice with water (and sugar, if used). Mix yogurt with cottage cheese and beat well to get rid of any lumps. Then add the lemon juice and water mixture. Mix well and pour over salad.

Grated Zucchini Salad with Lime

Preparation time: 15 minutes
Serves 2-4

1 lb. zucchini
juice of 1 lime (or lemon)
1 red bell pepper, grated
1 clove garlic, crushed
lettuce

Grate the zucchini finely. Mix with the lime (or lemon) juice and grated pepper. Add crushed garlic. Allow the flavors to blend a little before serving on a bed of lettuce.

Hungarian Tomato Salad

Preparation time: 15 minutes

whole tomatoes
lettuce
chopped chives

Dressing:
yogurt
lemon juice
flaxseed oil
grated horseradish

Skin the tomatoes by dipping them in boiling water for a minute. Make the dressing. Place the whole, skinned tomatoes on the lettuce leaves and cover with the dressing. Garnish with chopped chives.

Jumbo Salad

Preparation time: 20 minutes*
*Does not include presoaking
Serves 4-6

variety of shredded lettuce leaves
and salad greens, bite-sized and shredded

Any, or all, of the following:
tomato, chopped
green (or red) bell pepper, chopped
green onions, finely sliced
carrot
beet
radish, finely sliced
fennel, finely sliced
grape halves
lemon juice
flaxseed oil
dried dill weed
raisins, presoaked

Gradually build up the salad, beginning with the bite-sized shredded lettuce leaves and salad greens. Add any, or all, of the ingredients listed above. Presoak the raisins (soak overnight in cold water, or pour boiling water over them and leave for a couple of hours until plump). Sprinkle on top of the salad. Grate the carrot and/or beet and place to one side of the salad. (If you put it all on top, it tends to "smother" the salad.) Pour on the lemon juice and flaxseed oil. Sprinkle with dill. Serve with rice, oven-cooked and sliced potatoes or boiled small new potatoes.

Minted Apple and Celery Salad

Preparation time: 15 minutes*
* Does not include presoaking
Serves 2

1 red eating apple

apple cider vinegar
1 stalk of celery
raisins, presoaked
mint leaves
lettuce

Cut and core the apple and chop into bite-sized chunks. Mix with a little apple cider vinegar (diluted with water, if desired). Chop the celery and add, with the presoaked raisins (soak overnight in cold water, or pour boiling water over them and leave for a couple of hours until plump), to the apple and apple cider vinegar. Take the mint leaves and tear into small pieces. Add to the dish and serve on a bed of lettuce. (Leave for a little while before serving so the flavors have time to mix.)

Variation: Yogurt can be mixed with the apple cider vinegar for the dressing.

Orange, Chicory and Watercress Salad

Preparation time: 15 minutes
Serves 2-4

1 orange
2 heads of chicory
1 bunch of watercress

Dressing:
1 tbsp. flaxseed oil
1/2 tbsp. apple cider vinegar (or lemon juice)
1 clove garlic, crushed
1 green onion
parsley
chives
dill
fennel
mint

Peel the orange and split into segments. Separate the chicory leaves and arrange like the spokes of a wheel around a large dish. Put the watercress and orange in the middle. Combine all the dressing ingredients in a jug and stir vigorously. (If you have no fresh herbs, use a generous pinch of dried herbs.) Pour over the salad and serve immediately.

Radish, Apple and Celery Salad

*Preparation time: 15 minutes**
** Does not include presoaking*
Serves 2

radishes
green apples
celery
raisins
lettuce

Dressing:
1 tbsp. apple cider vinegar
1 tbsp. water
1 tsp. sugar (or honey)
1 or 2 cloves garlic, crushed
dill, chopped
yogurt

Chop the radishes, green apples and celery into small chunks. Presoak the raisins (soak overnight in cold water, or pour boiling water over them and leave for a couple of hours until plump) and add. For the dressing, mix together the apple cider vinegar, water, sugar (or honey), garlic and dill. Add enough yogurt to make a creamy dressing. Pour over the salad and serve on a bed of lettuce (include radicchio or red leaf, if available).

Variations: Use other herbs instead of dill, omit the yogurt or add some flaxseed oil.

Raw Turnip, Watercress and Orange Salad

Preparation time: 15 minutes
Serves 2

1 turnip
1 orange
watercress

Dressing:
orange juice
flaxseed oil

Peel and cut the turnip into matchstick-size pieces. Segment the orange and add to the turnip pieces. Add the watercress and toss in the dressing.

Rice Salad

Preparation time: 15 minutes
Serves 2

green bell pepper
red bell pepper
tomato
1 cup cooked brown rice

Dressing:
1 tbsp. flaxseed oil
1 tbsp. apple cider vinegar
1 clove garlic
sugar

Chop the peppers and tomato. Prepare the dressing, mix well and add the chopped peppers and tomato. Spoon onto the rice. Serve with a mixed green salad.

Romaine Lettuce with Yogurt Dressing

Preparation time: 10 minutes

Romaine lettuce
chives, chopped

Dressing:
yogurt
sugar
lemon juice
crushed garlic

Coarsely shred the lettuce. Pour on the dressing and sprinkle with chopped chives.

Salad Kebabs

Preparation time: 15 minutes

tomatoes
zucchinis
whole radishes
lettuce hearts
carrots

Dressing:
lemon juice
yogurt
flaxseed oil
herbs (mint, dill or parsley)

Thread on wooden skewers thinly sliced pieces of tomato, zucchini, whole radishes, lettuce hearts and raw carrot. Dip into the salad dressing before serving.

Salad Lorette

Preparation time: 10 minutes

cooked beets

celery stalks
lettuce

Dressing:
flaxseed oil
lemon juice

Thinly slice the beets and celery and mix with lettuce. Add dressing.

Spanish Salad

Preparation time: 15 minutes
Serves 2

onions
1 clove garlic
red bell peppers
tomatoes, sliced
parsley, chopped

Dressing:
flaxseed oil
1 tbsp. apple cider vinegar
1 tbsp. water
sugar (optional)

Thinly slice the onions and put into a bowl which has been rubbed over with a cut clove of garlic. Seed and slice the red peppers and lay them on top of the onion. Add a layer of sliced tomatoes. Crush the garlic and sprinkle on top. Pour over the dressing and sprinkle with chopped parsley.

Tomato and Zucchini Salad

Preparation time: 15 minutes
Serves 2

tomato
zucchini
green onion

beet
lettuce

Dressing:
flaxseed oil
yogurt
lemon juice

Chop the tomato and zucchini into chunks. Slice the green onion and add. Finely grate the raw beet (or chop cooked beet into chunks) and mix into the salad. Lay on a bed of lettuce. Pour over dressing.

Tomato Salad

Preparation time: 15 minutes
Serves 2

tomatoes
onion
1 tbsp. apple cider vinegar
1 tbsp. water
sugar (optional)
parsley, chopped
chives

Slice the tomatoes and spread out over a flat dish. Slice the onion and arrange the onion rings over the tomatoes. Mix the apple cider vinegar with water (and optional sugar, if used). Pour over the tomatoes and sprinkle with chopped parsley and chives.

Watercress, Endive and Grapefruit Salad

Preparation time: 10 minutes
Serves 2

watercress
endive (frisée or escarole, or both)
grapefruit
yogurt

Tear the watercress into smaller pieces, remove woody stems and put in a bowl with the endive leaves. Cut the grapefruit in half. Juice one half and segment the other half. Add the segments to salad leaves. Mix the grapefruit juice with yogurt and pour over the salad. Toss well and serve.

Zucchini Ribbon Salad

Preparation time: 10 minutes
Serves 2-4

3 large zucchinis
1 lb. tomatoes
6 green onions

Dressing:
2 tbsp. apple cider vinegar
pinch of sugar
2 tbsp. flaxseed oil
freshly chopped cilantro

Using a vegetable peeler or cheese slicer, cut the zucchinis lengthwise into thin ribbons, running along the side so the ribbons include the green skin. Place into a bowl. Quarter the tomatoes and thinly slice the onions. Add to the bowl. Toss in the dressing just before serving.

Soups

Apple and Fennel Soup

Preparation time: 15 minutes
Cooking time: 30-45 minutes
Serves 4

1 lb. potatoes
2 bulbs fennel
2 leeks
2 Granny Smith apples
1 tsp. sugar (optional)

1 tart eating apple

Peel and dice the potatoes, trim and chop the fennel, slice the leeks, and core and chop the apples into small pieces. Put these ingredients into a pot and cover with water. Bring to a boil, turn down the heat and simmer gently until potatoes and fennel are cooked. Purée (with electric blender or food mill). Add the chopped apples to the puréed soup. Serve immediately.

Variation: Omit apples, if you wish.

Argyll Soup

Preparation time: 10 minutes
Cooking time: 45 minutes
Serves 4

2 large carrots
2 large onions
4 sticks celery
1 lb. potatoes
2 cloves garlic
parsley

Slice the carrots, roughly chop the onions and slice the celery. Peel and chop the potatoes and crush the garlic. Put all into a large pot and cover with water. Bring to a boil. Turn down the heat and simmer gently for 45 minutes. Purée (with electric blender or food mill). Garnish with parsley and serve immediately.

Autumn Flame Soup

Preparation time: 15 minutes
Cooking time: 25 minutes
Serves 4

1 large onion
3 large cloves garlic
1 lb. squash (or pumpkin)
4 large red bell peppers

1 lb. tomatoes, chopped

thyme

fresh green herbs (2 small bay leaves, fresh parsley or cilantro)

Chop the onion and crush the garlic. Peel and chop the squash into small chunks. Seed the peppers and chop into small pieces. Put it all into a pot and cover with water. Bring to a boil. Turn down the heat and add the chopped tomatoes, thyme and bay leaves. Simmer gently for no longer than 20 minutes. Purée (with electric blender or food mill). Serve immediately, garnished with fresh green herbs of your choice.

Beet Soup

Preparation time: 15 minutes
Cooking time: 1 hour
Serves 4

2 medium beets, unpeeled

1 large onion

1 medium carrot

2 large tomatoes

red cabbage leaves, chopped

1 bay leaf

water

1 tbsp. apple cider vinegar

juice of 1/2 lemon

herbs

yogurt

parsley

Chop beets, onion, carrot and tomatoes, without peeling (except for the onion!). Put into a large pot. Add chopped cabbage leaves and bay leaf. Cover with water and add apple cider vinegar, lemon juice and herbs. Bring to a boil, then lower heat and simmer gently for about 1 hour. When cooked, purée (with electric blender or food mill), serve with a swirl of yogurt and garnish with parsley.

Cabbage Soup

Preparation time: 10 minutes
Cooking time: 40 minutes
Serves 2-4

1 small green (or white) cabbage
2 leeks
2 potatoes, peeled
2 onions
2 sticks celery
1 clove garlic
yogurt
parsley, chopped

Coarsely chop the vegetables. Put in a pot and cover with water. Bring to a boil, lower the heat and simmer until vegetables are tender. Purée (with electric blender or food mill). Serve hot with swirls of yogurt and garnished with chopped parsley.

Broccoli Floret Soup

Preparation time: 15 minutes
Cooking time: 35 minutes
Serves 2-4

1 medium onion
6 oz. potato
1 lb. broccoli
bay leaf
yogurt

Peel and chop the onion and potato. Trim the broccoli and cut into florets. Keep a few florets to one side and put the rest into a pot with the chopped onion, potato and bay leaf, and cover with water. Bring to a boil and simmer for 20 minutes. Add the other florets and simmer for an additional 10 minutes. Remove the bay leaf. Take the whole florets from the soup and put onto a hot plate. Put the rest of the soup through the food mill. Add the other cooked florets. Reheat the soup gently. Serve immediately with a swirl of yogurt.

Carrot and Orange Soup

Preparation time: 10 minutes
Cooking time: 40 minutes
Serves 2-4

1 lb. carrots
8 oz. onions
8 oz. potatoes
juice of 1 orange
a pinch of thyme

Chop the vegetables and put them into a pot with the orange juice and the thyme, and cover with water. Bring to a boil, then simmer until vegetables are tender. Purée (with electric blender or food mill).

Cauliflower Soup

Preparation time: 10 minutes
Cooking time: 40 minutes
Serves 2-4

1 large cauliflower
1 onion
1 celery stick
10 oz. yogurt
parsley, chopped

Trim the cauliflower and break into small florets. Chop the onion and slice the celery. Put into a pot and cover with water. Bring to a boil, lower the heat and simmer gently for 30 minutes. Purée (with electric blender or food mill). Stir in the yogurt. Reheat gently before serving. Garnish with chopped parsley.

Celery, Carrot and Apple Soup

Preparation time: 10 minutes
Cooking time: 45 minutes
Serves 2-4

1 lb. celery
1 lb. carrots
8 oz. sweet apples (Pink Lady or Gala)
dill (or lemon grass)
celery leaves, chopped

Slice the celery, dice the carrots and chop the apples. Put into a large pot and cover with water. Bring to a boil, lower the heat, add the dill (or lemon grass) and simmer for 40 minutes. Purée (with electric blender or food mill). Serve immediately and garnish with chopped celery leaves.

Celery Root and Swiss Chard Soup

Preparation time: 10 minutes
Cooking time: 40 minutes
Serves 2-4

1 small celery root
1 medium leek
2 oz. Swiss chard
apple cider vinegar (or lemon juice)
parsley

Scrub and chop the celery root and leek and tear the Swiss chard into small pieces. Put into a pot with apple cider vinegar (or lemon juice) and cover with water. Bring to a boil, turn down the heat and simmer until the vegetables are soft. Purée (with electric blender or food mill). Serve hot or cold and garnish with parsley.

Corn Chowder

Preparation time: 10 minutes
Cooking time: 45 minutes
Serves 2-4

3 sticks celery
1 large potato, peeled
1 large onion
1 large green bell pepper
1 bay leaf (or a pinch of ground bay leaf)
4 ears of corn
parsley, chopped

Dice the celery, potato and onion. Remove the seeds from the pepper and dice the flesh. Put into a pot with the bay leaf and cover with water. Simmer gently until the vegetables are almost cooked. Slice the corn from the cobs and add to the soup. Cook slowly until all the vegetables are soft but not broken (about 5 minutes.). Sprinkle with the chopped parsley and serve.

Potato, Cabbage and Dill Soup

Preparation time: 10 minutes
Cooking time: 40 minutes
Serves 2-4

1 medium potato, peeled
1 medium onion
1 medium leek
white cabbage, chopped
4 tsp. dried dill
chives, chopped

Chop the potato, onion and leek. Put into a pot with the chopped cabbage and cover with water. Bring to a boil, turn down the heat and add half the dill. Simmer gently until the potatoes are cooked. Purée (with electric blender or food mill). Add the rest of the dill and reheat gently. Garnish with chopped chives and serve immediately.

Potato Soup

Preparation time: 20 minutes
Cooking time: 1-1/2 to 2 hours
Serves 4-6

1 large onion
1/2 small celery knob
2 stalks celery
2 large potatoes
1 leek
parsley
2 quarts water

Dice all vegetables. Place vegetables, parsley and water in covered saucepan and bring to boil. Lower heat and cover. Simmer 1-1/2 to 2 hours. Mash through food mill.

Sweet and Sour Cabbage Soup

Preparation time: 10 minutes
Cooking time: 15 minutes
Serves 2-4

2 medium onions
1 medium white (or green) cabbage
2 cloves garlic, crushed
2 medium tomatoes
1 tbsp. sugar
juice of 1 large lemon
3 oz. raisins
1 qt. water

Slice the onion and sweat gently in a little water for a few minutes until it starts to soften. Cut the cabbage into thin strips and add to onion, mixing well. Add crushed garlic. Chop the tomatoes and add together with the sugar, lemon juice, raisins and water. Bring to a boil and simmer until the cabbage is al dente (about 10 minutes). Serve this hearty soup as a main dish with bread followed by fruit for dessert.

Tangy Tomato Soup

Preparation time: 10 minutes
Cooking time: 25 minutes
Serves 2-4

1 lb. tomatoes
1 carrot
1 stick celery
1 onion
1 red bell pepper
little orange juice
yogurt

Chop tomatoes, carrot, celery and onion. Seed pepper and chop. Put all into a large pot and cover with water. Bring to a boil, turn down the heat and simmer until vegetables are tender. Purée (with electric blender or food mill). Add the orange juice. Reheat gently. Add a swirl of yogurt before serving.

Tomato Soup with Potato and Onion

Preparation time: 20 minutes
Cooking time: 40 minutes
Serves 3-4

2 large tomatoes
1 medium onion
2 medium potatoes
1 tsp. wine vinegar
small bay leaf

Dice all vegetables. Place all ingredients in covered saucepan, cover with water and cook over low flame for 35-40 minutes. Mash through food mill and serve hot.

Vegetables and Potatoes

Baked Pepper and Tomato Salad

Preparation time: 15 minutes
Cooking time: 30 minutes
Serves 2-4

3 red bell peppers
6 large tomatoes
1 medium red onion
3 cloves garlic
juice of 1 large lemon
3 tbsp. fresh, chopped mint
flaxseed oil

Bake the peppers and tomatoes whole at 350° F (177° C) until somewhat cooked but still firm. Skin the peppers and tomatoes, chop roughly and place in a serving dish. Finely slice the onion and very thinly slice the garlic. Add to the mixture in the dish. Add the lemon and mint. Mix well. Sprinkle with a little flaxseed oil.

*Baked Potato and Parsnip Rosti**

* Rosti means "broiled" or "roasted" (i.e., top-browned)
Preparation time: 15 minutes
Cooking time: 1-1/4 hour
Serves 2

8 oz. parsnips
8 oz. potatoes
1 onion, finely chopped
2 tbsp. fresh chives, finely chopped
herbs
3-1/2 oz. yogurt
a little grated horseradish (optional)

Core the parsnips. Peel and coarsely grate the potatoes and parsnips into a large bowl. Add finely chopped onion, chives, herbs and yogurt. Mix until well combined. Put the vegetable mixture into a shallow dish and cover. Bake for 1 hour at 375° F (190° C). Remove the lid and bake a little longer until it begins to brown and the top is crispy. Serve with a crisp salad or a vegetable (or both).

Baked Potatoes

Preparation time: 5 minutes

Baked potatoes should be thoroughly washed, not scraped or peeled. Bake in a low oven at 300° F (149° C) for 2 or 2-1/2 hours or, alternatively, bake for 50 minutes to 1 hour at 350° F (177° C).

Baked Potato with Beet and Onion

Preparation time: 15 minutes
Cooking time: 1 hour

1 baking potato
1 large onion, peeled
beet, diced and cooked
yogurt
dill
1 tsp. flaxseed oil (optional)

Scrub the potato and place whole into a casserole dish with a large, peeled onion. Add a little water and bake until both are cooked. Chop the cooked onion and put into a saucepan with the diced, cooked beet. Heat through. Split open the potato and fill with the onion and beet mixture. Mix together the yogurt, dill and flaxseed oil (if using the flaxseed oil, wait until the potato is no longer steaming) and drizzle over the top. Serve with a green salad.

Baked Potato with Onion

Preparation time: 15 minutes
Cooking time: 1-1/2 hours

1 baking potato

1 onion
cooked beet
yogurt
dill

Bake the potato in its skin. Slice the onion and cook gently until beginning to soften. Dice the beet, add to the onion and warm through. When the potato is cooked, split it open and spoon in the beet mixture. Top with dollops of yogurt and sprinkle with dill. Serve with a green salad.

Baked Tomatoes

Preparation time: 10 minutes
Cooking time: 20 minutes
Serves 2

1 lb. tomatoes
1 clove garlic
1 medium onion
bread crumbs (or a handful of rolled oats)
dill
flaxseed oil

Slice the tomatoes and put into a baking dish. Crush the garlic, chop the onion and sprinkle over the tomatoes. Cover with bread crumbs (or rolled oats) and bake for about 20 minutes at 325° F (170° C). Just before serving, sprinkle with dill and flaxseed oil.

Beets

Bake at 300-350° F (149-177° C) or boil beets in their jackets.

Beets, Cooked and Creamed

Preparation time: 15 minutes
Cooking time: 60-75 minutes

3 beets, cooked and chopped

6 tbsp. yogurt
1 tbsp. fresh chives, snipped
2 tbsp. onion, finely chopped
parsley, finely chopped

Put cooked, chopped beets into a saucepan with the yogurt, chives and onion and heat gently. Put into serving dish and sprinkle with chopped parsley.

Beets with Horseradish

Preparation time: 10 minutes
Cooking time: 1 to 1-1/2 hours
Serves 2-4

6 beets
yogurt
2 tsp. horseradish
chives

Cook the beets until tender. Remove the skin and cut into quarters. Combine the yogurt and horseradish and pour over the beets. Garnish with chopped chives and serve immediately.

Bessarabian Nightmare

Preparation time: 15 minutes
Cooking time: 40 minutes
Serves 2

tomatoes
onions
red (or green) bell pepper, seeded
garlic, crushed
herbs
flaxseed oil

Skin the tomatoes. Slice the tomatoes, onions and peppers. Arrange in layers in an oven-proof dish. Sprinkle with crushed garlic and herbs.

Cook slowly, then chill and serve cold, adding a little flaxseed oil before serving. A strange name for a delicious dish!

Braised Cabbage

Preparation time: 15 minutes
Cooking time: 1 hour
Serves 2

1 lb. green cabbage
4 oz. carrots
4 oz. onion
2 sticks celery
dill seeds

Cut the cabbage into quarters. Remove the stalk, the core and any discolored leaves. Cook the cabbage in a little water in a saucepan for 10 minutes. Dice the carrots, onion and celery and put into a large oven-proof dish with very little water. Place the cabbage on top. Scatter with dill seeds. Bake covered for about 1 hour at 350° F (180° C) or until the vegetables are tender.

Braised Fennel with Orange and Tomato Sauce

Preparation time: 10 minutes
Cooking time: 30 minutes
Serves 2

1 medium head of fennel
1-1/2 lb. tomatoes
1 tbsp. tomato purée
juice of 1/2 orange
herbs
green fennel tops

Cut the fennel into quarters and remove the core. Cook gently for 8-10 minutes. Meanwhile, cook the tomatoes to a pulp and add the tomato purée, orange juice and herbs. Add the fennel and cook covered for 12-15 minutes. Garnish with fennel tops and serve.

Broccoli

Bake in a covered casserole in low oven at 300° F (149° C) with onions or a small amount of soup stock for 1-2 hours. Serve with tomato sauce.

Broccoli and Herbs

Preparation time: 20 minutes
Cooking time: 25 minutes
Serves 2

2 bunches of broccoli
4-6 cloves garlic
1/2 onion sliced
1/4 tsp. dill
1/4 cup soup stock

Peel the broccoli stems. Put garlic and onion in one pot and cook until onion becomes translucent. Add cut broccoli crowns and stems, dill and soup stock. Cook on low heat until broccoli is tender.

Broccoli, Green Beans and Pears

Preparation time: 5 minutes
Cooking time: 20 minutes
Serves 2

broccoli
green beans
2 pears

Dressing:
lemon juice (or apple cider vinegar)
flaxseed oil

Gently cook the broccoli and green beans. Allow to cool. Peel and chop the pears and put in a dish together with the broccoli and beans. Gently toss in dressing and serve with a baked potato and a mixed green salad.

Butternut Squash (Mashed)

Preparation time: 10 minutes
Cooking time: 35 minutes
Serves 2

butternut squash
1 small onion
yogurt

Peel and core chunks of butternut squash. Place in pan with one small onion. You will probably not need cooking water as the butternut squash is a "wet" vegetable. Simmer until done. Mash with enough yogurt to make smooth.

Cabbage and Tomato Hot Pot

Preparation time: 15 minutes
Cooking time: 35 minutes
Serves 2

1 small cabbage
1 onion
1 dessert apple
4 large tomatoes, skinned
yogurt
bread crumbs
parsley, chopped

Cook the cabbage gently in water until cooked but still crisp. Chop the onion, apple and skinned tomatoes and cook gently until they form a thick purée. Shred the cabbage and add to the purée. Turn into a casserole dish. Mix the yogurt with the bread crumbs and sprinkle over the top. Top-brown under the broiler to heat a little. Sprinkle with chopped parsley and serve immediately.

Carrot and Leek Bake

Preparation time: 10 minutes
Cooking time: 1-2 hours
Serves 2-4

1 lb. carrots
4 or 5 small leeks
2 medium oranges
handful of raisins

Dice or slice the carrots and slice the leeks. Put into a baking dish with the raisins. Add the juice of two oranges. Bake in a medium oven at 325° F (170° C) for 1 to 2 hours until done. If you wish, you can thicken the orange juice with corn starch to make a sauce. (Organic corn starch may be used occasionally.) Serve with a baked potato.

Carrot and Tomato Casserole

Preparation time: 15 minutes
Cooking time: 1 hour
Serves 2

8 oz. tomatoes
1/2 tbsp. chopped fresh sage (or 1/2 tsp. dried sage)
2 medium onions
1 lb. carrots

Slice or chop the tomatoes and put a layer into the bottom of a casserole dish. Add some sage. Slice the onions and place a layer on top of the tomatoes. Add another sprinkling of sage. Slice the carrot and place on top, finishing with a layer of tomato mixed with the last of the sage. Place the casserole in the oven and bake for 1 hour at 350° F (180° C) until the carrots are tender. Serve with a mixed green salad and a baked potato.

Carrots and Honey

Preparation time: 10 minutes
Cooking time: 45 minutes
Serves 1-2

carrots
soup stock
1/2 tsp. honey

Cut off the ends of the carrots and slice. Do not peel or scrape. Stew in a small amount of soup stock for 45 minutes or until tender. During the last 5 to 10 minutes of stewing, add honey for slight flavoring.

Cauliflower

Preparation time: 10 minutes
Cooking time: 45 minutes

cauliflower
2-3 tomatoes

Break cauliflower into sections. Add tomatoes, sliced and cut into chunks. Stew together for approximately 45 minutes (or until tender) on low heat.

Cauliflower and Carrot Sauce

Preparation time: 20 minutes
Cooking time: 50 minutes

1 small cauliflower
3 carrots
flaxseed oil

Separate the cauliflower florets, place them in a baking dish with a little water and cook at 250° F (121° C) for 40 minutes or until soft. When ready, drain off the water. At the same time, simmer the carrots on low heat with enough water until they are soft. Blend carrots in blender with the flaxseed oil. Pour sauce over the cooked cauliflower and place in warm oven at 250-300° F (121-149° C) (turned off) for 5-10 minutes before serving.

Chard Rolls, Stuffed

Preparation time: 40 minutes
Cooking time: 30 minutes

1/2 onion, sliced
6 medium potatoes
4 carrots
3 large cloves garlic, minced
1 bunch of chard

Cook onions and potatoes in one pot. In another pot, cook carrots and garlic. When done, purée (with electric blender or food mill) each potful separately, then mix together. Put chard leaves in very hot water, being sure not to overcook. Spread each leaf and remove tough center stem. Place purée in center of each leaf and roll tightly. Display on tray and serve with tomato sauce made with tomatoes, onion, garlic and small potato, which have been cooked and puréed.

Cooked Sweet Potato and Beet Salad

Preparation time: 10 minutes
Cooking time: 30 minutes
Serves 2

1 large (or 2 small) sweet potatoes
a few cooked small beets, sliced
arugula (or lettuce) leaves

Dressing:
yogurt
lemon juice
flaxseed oil
dill weed, dried or fresh

Cook the sweet potatoes gently in their skins until done. Allow to cool. Cut into slices and place the sweet potato and beet slices overlapping on a plate of arugula (or lettuce) leaves. Drizzle on the dressing and serve immediately.

Corn

Preparation time: 5 minutes

Corn may be baked in the husk wrapped in foil. Bake in low oven at 300° F (149° C) for 1 hour. If husked, place in boiling water for approximately 7 minutes.

Corn on the Cob Packets

Preparation time: 5 minutes
Cooking time: 1 hour
Serves 1-2

1 or 2 corn cobs
flaxseed oil
parsley, chopped

Leave the corn in its outer leaves and wrap in baking foil. Bake at 350° F (180° C) for about 1 hour. When cooked, peel back the leaves and allow to cool. Pour on some flaxseed oil to which some chopped parsley has been added. Serve as an appetizer or a side dish.

Corn with Mixed Vegetables

Preparation time: 15 minutes
Cooking time: 1 hour
Serves 2

2 ears of corn
3 stalks of celery
2 carrots
2 zucchinis squash

Husk the corn and cut the kernels off. Slice the other vegetables into small pieces. Put the corn in a baking dish and add the vegetables. Bake at 200° F (93° C) for 1 hour.

Corn with Orange Juice

Preparation time: 10 minutes

2 ears of corn
1 glass of orange juice

Husk the corn, cut off the kernels and put it in a baking dish with a lid. Bake at 250° F (121° C) until soft (approximately 25-30 minutes). Pour the corn juice off and add the orange juice. Let set 5 to 10 minutes before serving.

Creamed Corn

Preparation time: 20 minutes
Cooking time: 1-1/2 hours
Serves 2-3

3 ears of corn
1 green bell pepper, sliced

Husk corn and cut off the kernels. Put kernels from 2 ears in a blender and blend. Add the kernels from the third ear to the blended corn. Place in a baking dish and put the sliced green pepper on top and bake in the oven at 200-250° F (93-121° C) for 1-1/2 hours.

Creamed Green Beans

Preparation time: 5 minutes
Cooking time: 15 minutes
Serves 2

10 oz. whole green beans
yogurt
2 oz. onion, finely chopped

Cook the beans gently. Just before the beans are ready, gently heat the yogurt with the chopped onion. Put the beans into a warm serving dish and pour on the yogurt dressing.

Creamy Cabbage

Preparation time: 10 minutes
Cooking time: 30 minutes
Serves 2

white cabbage
1 small onion
2 tbsp. yogurt
1 tsp. dried dill tops, chopped (or crushed dill seeds)

Shred the cabbage and chop the onion. Add a little water to cook. When cooked and tender, add the yogurt mixed with the dill tops (or seeds).

Eggplant, Baked

Preparation time: 15 minutes
Cooking time: 2 hours
Serves 2

soup stock
1 onion, chopped
1 eggplant, sliced
2 tomatoes, sliced and skinned

Put some soup stock in bottom of large covered baking dish. Add onion, eggplant and tomatoes in layers. Cover and bake in a low oven at 300° F (149° C) for 2 hours.

Eggplant Fan

Preparation time: 15 minutes
Cooking time: 45 minutes
Serves 2

1 large onion

1 large eggplant
1 large firm, ripe tomato
thyme and marjoram
1 small clove garlic, chopped

Slice the onion into rings and cook gently in a thick-bottomed saucepan while preparing the other ingredients. Cut eggplant into 4 or 5 lengthwise slices, stopping 3/4 inch from either end. Slice the tomato into twice as many slices as there are cuts in the eggplant. Arrange the eggplant on top of the onions in a fan shape, and fill the cuts with the tomato slices. Sprinkle with herbs and chopped garlic. Cover and cook gently, on top of the stove, or bake gently in a low oven at 300° F (149° C) until the eggplant is soft.

Eggplant Salad

Preparation time: 15 minutes
Cooking time: 1 hour
Serves 2
1 eggplant
1 small onion
parsley
2 tomatoes
1-1/2 tbsp. vinegar
a little flaxseed oil

Bake the eggplant for about 1 hour at 350° F (180° C). Chop the onion and parsley and slice the tomatoes. Combine with the cooked eggplant. Add the vinegar and flaxseed oil.

Eggplant, Stewed

Preparation time: 20 minutes
Cooking time: 30 minutes
Serves 2

1 eggplant, cut into cubes
2 onions, chopped

3 tomatoes, peeled and chopped

Combine all ingredients in a stew pot. Stew approximately 30 minutes (until tender). Do not add water.

Fancy Garlic Potatoes

Preparation time: 5 minutes
Cooking Time: 1-1/2 to 2 hours

potatoes
flaxseed oil
garlic, crushed

Cut the potatoes into slices, not quite through to the base. Put into a casserole dish with only enough water to cover the bottom. Cook in the top of the oven at 325° F (170° C) for 1-1/2 to 2 hours or at 350° F (180° C) for 1 hour. Mix together the flaxseed oil and crushed garlic. Put the potatoes onto a serving dish and, when slightly cooled, pour on the dressing. Serve immediately.

Fennel Treat

Preparation time: 15 minutes
Cooking time: 1-2 hours
Serves 2

1 fennel bulb
1 large tomato, cut into 1/4-inch slices
2-3 cloves garlic, peeled and sliced thinly

Cut off stalks and leaves from fennel. Slice bulb in half lengthwise to give two flat halves. Rinse under running water to remove sand and put them in a baking dish with cut side up. Cover halves with tomato slices and place garlic slices on top of tomatoes. Cover the dish and bake at 250° F (121° C) for 1 to 2 hours. Serve with a baked potato and a salad of grated carrots on a bed of pretty greens.

Festive Broccoli (or Festive Green Beans)

Preparation time: 25 minutes
Cooking time: 45 minutes
Serves 2-3

1 large head broccoli (or 3-1/2 cups sliced green beans)
1 small onion, diced
1 clove garlic, minced
1 medium sweet red (or yellow) bell pepper, cut in strips
2 tsp. lemon juice (optional)
1/4 tsp. dried (or 1 tsp. fresh) dill weed

Select dark green head of broccoli with no yellowing. Cut into spears, peeling tougher stalks at base. Place onion and garlic in pot. Cover and stew on low flame for 45 minutes or until tender. Add pepper strips for the last 20 to 25 minutes of cooking. Add lemon juice just before serving (lemon will discolor broccoli if added during cooking). Sprinkle vegetables with dill and serve.

French Bean (Green Bean) Salad

Preparation time: 5 minutes
Cooking time: 10 minutes
Serves 2

French beans (green beans)
small onion, chopped
flaxseed oil
apple cider vinegar (or lemon juice)
parsley
chives

Cook the beans gently until just tender. Drain and add the chopped onion. Put into a serving dish and toss in the flaxseed oil and apple cider vinegar (or lemon juice). Add herbs and serve.

Fruited Red Cabbage

Preparation time: 10 minutes*
* Does not include soaking
Cooking time: 15 minutes
Serves 2

4 oz. raisins
4 oz. dried apricots, chopped
1 small red cabbage
2 dessert apples, cored and chopped
apple cider vinegar
a little sugar

Presoak the raisins and apricots (soak overnight in cold water, or pour boiling water over them and leave for a couple of hours until plump). Shred the red cabbage and sweat in a little water until slightly softened. Add raisins, chopped apricots and cored, chopped dessert apples. Toss in apple cider vinegar, to which a little water and sugar have been added. Pile into a bowl and serve with a baked potato.

Gerson Gardener's Pie*

*A bit like Shepherd's Pie but with vegetables instead of meat
Preparation time: 30 minutes
Cooking time: 2-1/2 hours
Serves 2-3

Topping:
1 lb. potatoes
12 oz. celery root (or sweet potato or onion)

Peel the potato and other vegetable and cut into small chunks. Add water but only about 1/2 to 2/3 the height of the vegetables. Bring to a boil and reduce to a simmer. Cook slowly until all the water is gone and the vegetables are soft, and mash. If there is a little water left in the pan, beat it into the mash mixture.

Filling:
1 small onion (or a few shallots)

2 cloves garlic, crushed

8 oz. carrots, sliced, or chipped or diced (but not diced too thickly)

8 oz. zucchini, cut into half slices, not too thin

8 oz. leeks, trimmed and sliced

2 tomatoes, skinned and chopped

1-2 tbsp. chopped parsley

herbs to taste

2 oz. bread crumbs

Prepare vegetables and put them into a saucepan in the order listed above. Cook the vegetables very gently. You may need to use a simmer plate. This could take 1 to 1-1/2 hours. Prepare topping and bread crumbs. When vegetables are cooked, stir in bread crumbs and pour the mixture into a pie plate. Top with mashed potatoes. Drag a fork over the top to decorate and bake for about 45 to 60 minutes at 350° F (180° C). Place pie plate on baking sheet in case of leakage. Serve with green vegetables and salad.

Variations: Change the contents of the pie by adding green beans, peas and/or corn when in season. Jerusalem artichokes would be also good. You could leave the leeks out of the pie and purée them (with electric blender or food mill) to add to the topping instead of the sweet potato, onion or celery root.

Gerson Roast Potatoes

Preparation time: 5 minutes
Cooking time: 1 hour

1 baking potato

Cut a baking potato in half (or, if very large, into quarters). Score across the cut surface with a knife. Put into a casserole dish with a little water to just cover the bottom. Put lid on and bake in a hot oven at 400-425° F (204-218° C) for 1 hour. Before serving, remove the lid and leave to slightly brown.

Glazed Beets

Preparation time: 25 minutes
Cooking time: 1-1/2 hours
Serves 6 to 8

9 large beets

Scrub beets and boil in 2 to 3 inches of water until tender for 1 to 1-1/2 hours. Add more water if needed. Peel in cold water. Slice or cut into bite-sized pieces.

Glaze:
2/3 cup fresh orange juice
1 tsp. cornstarch
1-1/2 tsp. apple cider vinegar
1 tsp. honey (or sugar)

Combine ingredients for glaze. Cook over low flame until thick. Add beets and mix well.

   Variation: Use 1/2 cup apple juice and 3 tsp. lemon juice in place of orange Juice.

Glazed Carrots and Turnips with Garlic

Preparation time: 10 minutes
Cooking time: 30 minutes
Serves 2

8 oz. carrots
8 oz. turnips

Dressing:
1 tbsp. lemon juice
1 clove garlic, crushed
flaxseed oil

Gently cook the carrots and turnips. Cut into thin slices and put into a serving dish. Pour on the dressing and garnish with cilantro or dill.

Glazed Carrots with Herbs and Lemon

Preparation time: 5 minutes
Cooking time: 30 minutes
Serves 2

1 lb. carrots
1 tsp. sugar
a little water
1 tbsp. lemon juice
mint
rosemary
parsley
flaxseed oil

Gently cook the carrots whole. When beginning to soften, remove from pan and cut into 2-inch sticks. Return to the saucepan with the sugar and a little water. Heat until the sugar is dissolved, the water has been absorbed and the carrots are cooked. Add the lemon juice and herbs and heat for an additional 2 minutes. Place on a warm serving dish, add flaxseed oil and serve immediately.

Glazed Carrots with Orange

Preparation time: 5 minutes
Cooking time: 30 minutes
Serves 2

1 lb. carrots
1 tbsp. sugar
juice of 1/2 orange
flaxseed oil

Gently cook the carrots whole. When beginning to soften, remove from the pan and cut into 2-inch sticks. Return to the saucepan with the sugar and orange juice. Heat until the sugar has been dissolved and the orange juice absorbed. Turn onto platter, add flaxseed oil and serve.

Green Beans in Honey and Tomato Sauce

Preparation time: 15 minutes
Cooking time: 20 minutes
Serves 2

1 lb. fine green beans

Sauce:
1 medium onion
2 cloves garlic
1 lb. tomatoes, roughly chopped
1 tsp. honey
herbs

Cut ends off the beans, cook until just tender and drain. To make the sauce, chop the onion and crush the garlic. Cook them both in a little water until just tender. When the onion is soft, add the roughly chopped tomatoes and bring to a boil. Simmer gently until sauce becomes fairly thick. Stir in the honey and herbs. Add the beans and allow to cool. Serve at room temperature.

Green Chard Rolls

Preparation time: 45 minutes
Cooking time: 2 hours

4 leaves of green chard
2 carrots
1/4 head broccoli
1/4 head cauliflower
2 small zucchini squash
1 ear of corn (cut kernels off)
1/2 cup uncooked rice

Sauce:
1-1/2 tomatoes
2 cloves garlic

Put the chard leaves in hot water long enough to wilt them so they will bend. Cut the broccoli, cauliflower, squash and corn into small pieces and put them in a pan with a little water to simmer. When cooked, drain the water off. Make a sauce in the blender with the tomatoes and garlic, and pour this sauce on top of the vegetables and uncooked rice. Place some of the vegetables/rice mixture in the center of each leaf and roll them up. Put these in a baking dish with a lid and bake in the oven at 250° F (121° C) for 1 to 1-1/2 hours.

Green Peppers

Preparation time: 10 minutes
Cooking time: 30 minutes
Serves 2-3

2-4 green peppers, sliced
2-4 onions, sliced

Stew in tightly covered pot for approximately 30 minutes. Do not add water.

Grilled Eggplant

Preparation time: 10 minutes
Cooking time: 20 minutes
Serves 1

1 eggplant
garlic
parsley, chopped
lemon (or lime) juice

Slice the eggplant lengthwise. Heat a griddle pan (preferably a "ridged" pan). When the pan is hot, turn down the heat, place the slices of egg-plant on the griddle and allow them to cook slowly. Turn over the slices and repeat. Before serving, squeeze garlic over the slices, sprinkle with chopped parsley and drizzle lemon (or lime) juice over them. This is a good main course for lunch served with new potatoes.

Variations: You can do the same thing with large slices of peppers, halves of onions or zucchini halved lengthwise.

Leek and Potato Bake

Preparation time: 15 minutes
Cooking time: 40 minutes
Serves 2

1 lb. potatoes
1 small leek
fine oats (put some regular rolled oats in the blender)

Parboil the potatoes in their skins until they are hot through and just beginning to soften. Very thinly slice the leek (using the white section only). Peel the potatoes and coarsely grate them. Mix in the leek. Put into a shallow baking dish (sprinkled at the bottom with fine oats to prevent sticking). Cook on the top shelf of the oven at 350° F (180° C) until beginning to show signs of browning. (Don't leave it for too long or it will dry out.) Serve with either cooked vegetables or a green salad and tomatoes.

Leeks (or Zucchini) à la Grecque

Preparation time: 10 minutes
Cooking time: 30 minutes
Serves 2

1 lb. leeks (or zucchini)
3 tomatoes, chopped (optional)
juice of 1 lemon
bay leaf
thyme
coriander seeds

Slice the leeks (or zucchini) into 1-inch pieces. Cook gently with chopped tomatoes (if used), lemon juice, bay leaf, thyme and coriander seeds. Serve hot or cold.

Lima Beans and Zucchini

Preparation time: 15 minutes
Cooking time: 20 minutes
Serves 1-2

1 large onion
1 clove garlic
1/2 cup soup stock
1 cup fresh lima beans
3 cups zucchini
4 medium tomatoes
1/2 tsp. cornstarch
4 sprigs fresh parsley
dash of thyme (or sage, or a pinch of dried parsley)

Mix together all ingredients except herbs. Simmer about 15 minutes (until tender). Thicken with cornstarch mixed with a little water. Just before serving, add herbs.

Lyonnaise Potatoes

Preparation time: 5 minutes
Cooking Time: 1 to 1-1/2 hours
Serves 2

1 lb. potatoes
1 large onion
2 tbsp. of water
flaxseed oil
garlic, crushed

Thickly slice the potatoes and onion. Arrange the potato slices in an oven-proof dish with a slice of onion between each potato slice. Pour on the water. Bake in oven at 300-350° F (149-177° C) until well done and beginning to brown. Allow to cool slightly, then pour on the flaxseed oil and crushed garlic. Serve immediately.

Mashed Carrot and Potato Bake

Preparation time: 10 minutes
Cooking time: 1 hour

carrots
potatoes

Cook the carrots and potatoes gently until just tender. Mash them and pile into an oven-proof dish. Decorate with diagonal fork marks and put into a hot oven at 400-425° F (204-218° C) to brown.

Mashed Potatoes

Preparation time: 20 minutes
Cooking time: 40 minutes

potatoes
1 small onion
yogurt

Peel and cube potatoes. Place in pan with one small onion and enough water to bring to a boil. Simmer until done (when there is no water left). Mash with enough yogurt to make smooth.

Mashed Potatoes and Chard

Preparation time: 15 minutes
Cooking time: 25 minutes
Serves 4

1 bunch green (or red) chard
4-5 tbsp. water (or soup stock)
3 large (or 4 medium) potatoes
6-8 oz. yogurt

Shred the chard and put in pan. Add water (or soup stock) and start to boil. When boiling, turn down to simmer. Meanwhile, peel potatoes, cube and place on top of the chard. Let simmer until potatoes are soft and done. Remove any remaining water and add yogurt. Mash all together. Add a little more yogurt if the mixture is too dry.

Variation: The same recipe can be used with kale. When using kale, strip out central stems before shredding into pan.

Mashed Potatoes Gerson Style

Preparation time: 10 minutes
Cooking time: 35 minutes

potatoes, peeled and cut into pieces
onion, peeled and chopped small

Place potatoes and onions in a pot. Add just enough water to reach the vegetables half-way up. Cover, bring to boil and simmer until potatoes are cooked. (Most of the cooking water will probably be gone.) Mash potatoes and onions using some (or all) of the cooking water. If not enough moisture, add some soup stock.

Variations: Add any herb of your choice, finely chopped. Parsley is very good; mint and dill will also work.

Oven-Browned Potatoes

Preparation time: 5-10 minutes

potatoes

Cut the potatoes like French fries (or in small cubes, or in thin slices) and brown on an oven tray in the oven. They will brown at a surprisingly low heat (300° F or 149° C), if left in long enough. Depending on the variety of potato, they can brown very quickly and puff up at high heat (425° F or 218° C). They can also be browned under the broiler, but watch them to avoid burning. This is meant to be an occasional treat!

Parsley Potatoes

potatoes
parsley, chopped
flaxseed oil

Boil several potatoes in their skins until done. Remove the peel and roll in some chopped parsley after slightly brushing with flaxseed oil.

Parsnips and Sweet Potatoes

Preparation time: 10 minutes
Cooking time: 40 minutes
Serves 2-4

1 lb. parsnips
1 lb. sweet potatoes
sprig of fresh rosemary

Cut the parsnips and sweet potatoes into wedges, leaving the skins intact. Put into a baking dish with a little water to cover the bottom. Add a sprig of rosemary. Cover and bake in a medium oven at 325° F (170° C) until just cooked. Serve with a baked potato.

Patate alla Francesca

Preparation time: 5 minutes
Cooking time: 40 minutes

new potatoes
tomatoes
fresh rosemary sprigs
garlic

Bake new potatoes in a covered dish at 300-350° F (149-177° C) with chopped or sliced tomatoes, fresh rosemary sprigs and plenty of garlic. Serve with lemon wedges and a green salad.

Piemontese Peppers

Preparation time: 10 minutes
Cooking time: 1 hour
Serves 2

2 tomatoes
2 red bell peppers

2 cloves garlic, sliced
herbs

Skin the tomatoes. Halve the peppers and remove the seeds (but not the stalks). Place the peppers skin-side down in a baking dish. Place slices of garlic inside each pepper half and top each with half a skinned tomato. Bake covered at 350° F (180° C) until tender and sweet (about 1 hour). Serve hot or cold, sprinkled with herbs.

Potato and Celery Root Lyonnaise

Preparation time: 15 minutes
Cooking Time: 1-1/2 to 2 hours
Serves 2

1 small to medium onion
1 small to medium celery root, scrubbed (and, if necessary, peeled)
1 medium potato, scrubbed

Slice all the ingredients thinly. Arrange in layers (onion, celery root and, potato) in a small soufflé dish. Add a very little amount of water. Bake for 1-1/2 to 2 hours at 325° F (170° C). The top layer will get crisp while the lower layers should be soft. Serve with green vegetable of your choice and a salad.

Potato Cakes

Preparation time: 25 minutes
Cooking time: 30 minutes
Serves 2-4

1 lb. potatoes
1 large carrot
1 green bell pepper
1 stick of celery
fine oats (put some regular rolled oats in the blender)

Parboil the potatoes in their skins until they are hot through and just beginning to soften. Put through the food mill. (This will also get rid of the skin.) Cut carrot into thin matchsticks. Chop the green pepper and celery. Add these to the potato purée and form into small cakes. Coat with oats and bake in the oven at 325° F (170° C) on a baking sheet sprinkled with fine oats to prevent sticking.

Potatoes and Carrots, Westphalian Style

Preparation time: 10 minutes
Cooking time: 35 minutes
Serves 4

6-8 small (or 4-5 large carrots) carrots
3 medium (or 2 large) potatoes
1 large onion
3-4 tbsp. of soup stock

Slice carrots into pan. Peel and slice potatoes and chop onion. Add all together in pan with soup stock. Let simmer until done, adding a bit more soup stock, if necessary. When done, no liquid should remain in pan.

Potatoes Anna

Preparation time: 20 minutes
Cooking time: 1 to 1-1/2 hours
Serves 2

onion, cooked
1 lb. potatoes
garlic, crushed
yogurt
parsley, finely chopped

Sweat the onions in a covered saucepan over very low heat for approximately 1 hour. Using a 10-inch flan (or quiche) tin with at least 1-inch sides, place a layer of sweated onions on the bottom of the tin. Sprinkle with a little water to stop the onions from sticking. Very thinly slice the potatoes and layer them in the dish on top of the onions. Sprinkle with crushed garlic and some of the yogurt. Add an additional two layers, again sprinkling with garlic and yogurt. Press down each layer and make sure the potatoes overlap each other very slightly so there are no spaces. Cover the dish (e.g., by using a base from a larger, loose-bottomed cake tin). Bake at 350° F (180° C) for about 1 to 1 to 1-1/2 hours or until the potatoes feel soft when pierced with a knife. Check the potatoes while cooking; if they look too dry, add a little more yogurt. To serve, turn the potato cake out of its dish and sprinkle with finely chopped parsley.

Potato Puffs

Preparation time: 5 minutes
Cooking time: 45-50 minutes

baking potato

Take a baking potato and cut it into 1/2-inch slices. Place the slices on the oven rack and, without any addition, bake at high heat (425° F (218° C)) to puff. Turn over and lower heat to 325° F (163° C) with oven door cracked open. Bake for another 20 minutes. The slices puff up and become crisp and tasty, almost like fried potatoes. Done when shiny brown on both sides. This is marginal food, so eat it occasionally.

Potato Salad

Preparation time: 10 minutes
Cooking time: 20 minutes
Serves 2

1 lb. small new potatoes
large sprig of mint
1 tbsp. fresh parsley

Dressing:
4 oz. yogurt
a little flaxseed oil
2 cloves garlic, crushed

Scrub the potatoes and put in a saucepan with a little water. Gently simmer until cooked but still firm. While the potatoes are still hot, slice them and put into a warm dish. Pour over the dressing. Finish by sprinkling fresh chopped mint and parsley.

Quick Bake Potatoes

Preparation time: 5 minutes
Cooking time: 1 hour

potatoes
flaxseed oil

Cut potatoes in half lengthwise and score cut surfaces with diagonal lines crossing each other (like lattice work). They will cook in about half the time (about 50 minutes) in the oven at 300-350° F (149-177° C); when cool enough, the surfaces can be coated with flaxseed oil.

Quick Tomatoes and Zucchini

Preparation time: 5 minutes
Cooking time: 30 minutes
Serves 2

2 medium tomatoes
1 clove garlic, crushed
1/4 to 1/2 tsp. sugar (optional)
1 medium zucchini

Slice the tomatoes and place in the bottom of a saucepan, along with the crushed garlic and sugar (if using). Slice the zucchini and place on top. Set on a gentle heat. When the tomatoes begin to cook, stir, cover and cook for about 20 minutes.

Ratatouille

Preparation time: 15 minutes
Cooking time: 1 hour
Serves 2-4

8 oz. onions
8 oz. green/red/yellow bell peppers

8 oz. eggplant
4 tomatoes
1 clove garlic
2 tsp. apple cider vinegar
marjoram

Slice the onions and place in a baking dish. Seed and thinly slice the peppers. Add to the dish. Cut the eggplants in quarters lengthwise and then into 1/4-inch slices and add. Chop the tomatoes and finely chop the garlic clove. Add to the dish together with the apple cider vinegar and a sprinkling of marjoram. Cook very gently in the oven at 325° F (170° C) until well done. Can also be cooked on top of the stove.

Red Cabbage

Preparation time: 25 minutes
Cooking time: 1 hour
Serves 2-3

1/2 red cabbage, shredded
3 tsp. vinegar
3 large onions, chopped
2 bay leaves
a little soup stock
3 apples, peeled and grated
1 tsp. sugar

Combine cabbage, vinegar, onions, bay leaves and soup stock in a pan. Stew over low heat for approximately 1 hour. At the 1/2-hour mark, add apples and sugar.

Red Cabbage and Apple Casserole

Preparation time: 15 minutes
Cooking time: 1-1/2 hours
Serves 2

medium red cabbage
apples (cooking or green)

juice of 1 orange

apple cider vinegar

maple syrup

Shred the red cabbage and slice the apple. Place layers of red cabbage and apple in a casserole dish. Pour over the orange juice, apple cider vinegar and maple syrup. Cover with a tight-fitting lid and bake at 350° F (180° C) for about 1-1/2 hours or until tender. Stir and serve. Almost better as a reheated leftover!

Red Kuri Squash with Vegetables

Preparation time: 15 minutes
Cooking time: 30 minutes
Serves 2-4

1 red kuri squash

1 tbsp. water

1 small sweet potato, cooked

1 small zucchini, cooked

1 red (or green) bell pepper, cooked

1 tomato, peeled

onion (or garlic) powder

fresh herbs

Cut the red kuri squash in half. This is easily done with a very sharp, pointed knife. Scoop out the seeds, leaving the rest of the red flesh intact. Stand upright in an oven-proof dish to which the water has been added. Cover and bake at 300-350° F (149-177° C) until cooked (about 30 minutes; test by inserting a knife into the flesh). If there is enough room, the other vegetables could be cooked in the same dish. Otherwise, bake them in a separate dish in the same way, or cook them gently on top of the stove in a saucepan. When cooked, pile the vegetables into the squash halves. Sprinkle with onion (or garlic) powder or fresh herbs. Serve with a colorful mixed salad.

Roasted Zucchini and Pepper Salad

Preparation time: 10 minutes
Cooking time: 30 minutes
Serves 2

1 lb. small zucchini
2 red bell peppers
yogurt
3 tbsp. mint, roughly chopped

Dressing:
2 tbsp. lemon juice
2 cloves garlic, crushed
flaxseed oil

Cut the ends off the zucchini and cut in half lengthwise. Seed the peppers and cut into quarters. Put the zucchini and peppers skin-side up on a baking tray. Bake in oven at 325° F (170° C) for about 1/2 hour. When cooked and tender, cool slightly and cut into 1-inch lengths. Put into a serving dish, pour on the dressing and add the chopped mint. Serve with a smattering of cottage cheese (unsalted and uncreamed or fat-free).

Rolled Chard Parcels

Preparation time: 10 minutes
Cooking time: 30 minutes

chard leaves
green onions
snow peas
asparagus
broccoli
julienne of carrots
red chard stems

Set aside the chard leaves. Gently cook the green onions, snow peas, asparagus, broccoli, carrots and red chard stems in very little water and then chop them. Blanch the chard leaves. Fill with the cooked vegetable medley and form into "packets." Cook briefly in the oven at 300-350° F (149-177° C) for a few minutes until heated through. Serve hot or cold.

Root Vegetable Rosti*

* Rosti means "broiled" or "roasted" (i.e., top-browned)
Preparation time: 10 minutes
Cooking time: 1 hour
Serves 2

1 small onion
8 oz. potatoes
4 oz. carrots
4 oz. swede (rutabaga)
dill

Thinly slice the onion and cook by "sweating" in a little water. Meanwhile, gently cook the potatoes, carrots and swede (rutabaga). Drain thoroughly and, when cool enough to handle, coarsely grate into a bowl. Stir in the softened onion and dill. Put the mixture into an oven-proof dish. Bake for about 1/2 hour in the top of the oven at 350° F (180° C) or until cooked and slightly browning. Serve immediately.

Sauté of Sweet Potatoes

Preparation time: 15 minutes
Cooking time: 20 minutes
Serves 2-4

4 medium sweet potatoes
juice of 1 orange
a little sugar
flaxseed oil

Cook the sweet potatoes in their skins until just cooked. Allow to cool slightly, then cut into cubes. Put orange juice and sugar into a saucepan with the sweet potatoes. Heat gently but don't let the mixture boil. Put into a serving dish and allow to cool a little. Add the flaxseed oil, toss and serve immediately with fresh parsley (or chives) and a green salad.

Scalloped Potatoes (Without Yogurt)

Preparation time: 15 minutes
Cooking time: 1-2 hours

1 onion
potatoes
tomato, sliced
marjoram and/or thyme

Place a whole chopped onion in the bottom of a glass baking dish. Slice potatoes and place one layer on top of the onion. Add a layer of sliced tomato on top, then another layer of sliced or chopped onion. Sprinkle with a dash of marjoram and/or thyme and bake in a low oven at 300° F (149° C) for 1 to 2 hours or until done.

Scalloped Potatoes (With Yogurt)

Preparation time: 15 minutes
Cooking time: 1 to 1-1/2 hours
Serves 2

1 lb. potatoes
1 small onion
1 clove garlic
yogurt

Cook the potatoes gently until just cooked but firm. Slice thinly. Finely chop the onion and garlic. Arrange the slices of potato, layered with onion and garlic, in a pie dish. Pour over the yogurt and bake at 350° F (180° C) for 1 to 1-1/2 hours or until well cooked and beginning to brown on top.

Spinach

Preparation time: 10 minutes
Cooking time: 20 minutes

spinach
onions, chopped

After cutting off roots, wash spinach 3 to 4 times. Put in large, tightly covered pot that has a layer of chopped onions on the bottom of the pan. Do not add water. Stew over a low flame until spinach wilts. Pour off excess juice. Serve chopped with slice of lemon.

Spinach (or Chard) with Tomato Sauce

Preparation time: 15 minutes
Cooking time: 15 minutes

spinach (or chard)
lemon grass
sprig of rosemary
allspice (optional)

Cook the spinach (or chard) with some lemon grass and a sprig of rosemary. Add a pinch of allspice, if desired. Thinly cut the ribs of the spinach (or chard) and cook the leaves. Serve with tomato sauce.

Stuffed Eggplant

Preparation time: 20 minutes
Cooking time: 1 hour
Serves 2

1 eggplant
4 oz. tomatoes
1 medium onion
1 clove garlic, crushed
1 tbsp. fresh chopped parsley

Place the whole eggplant in a large saucepan and cover with boiling water. Let stand for 10 minutes, then plunge into cold water. Meanwhile, in another saucepan, very gently cook the tomatoes for 5 minutes. Press through sieve to get rid of the skins and set aside the pulp. Cut the cooled eggplants in half lengthwise. Scoop out the pulp, leaving a 1/2-inch thick outer shell. Chop the eggplant pulp and set aside. Place the eggplant shells in a shallow baking dish with just a little water in the bottom to prevent sticking. Bake for 30 minutes at 350° F (180° C). Sauté onion and crushed garlic in a small amount of boiling water until tender. Stir in the parsley. Add the sieved tomato pulp and chopped eggplant pulp, and cook for 20 minutes on moderate heat until it thickens. Spoon this mixture into the cooked eggplant shells. Keep warm in the oven until serving, or leave to cool and serve cold.

Stuffed Mixed Vegetables

Preparation time: 25 minutes
Cooking time: 30 minutes
Serves 2-4

1 zucchini
1 eggplant
2 small onions, chopped
garlic, crushed
marjoram
1 green (or red) bell pepper
soup stock

Cut the zucchini and eggplant in half, scoop out the pulp of the eggplant (carefully leaving a shell) and cook with the onion, crushed garlic and marjoram. Cut the peppers in half and take out the seeds. Stuff the eggplant, zucchini and peppers with the mixture and put in a shallow baking dish on a layer of onion rings. Bake at 300-350° F (149-177° C) until the pepper is done. Add a little soup stock if the dish seems to be getting dry. Serve with tomato sauce.

Stuffed Pepper

Preparation time: 10 minutes
Cooking time: 50 minutes
Serves 1

red (or green) bell pepper
leftover mixed, chopped vegetables
tomatoes, sliced

Halve the pepper and seed it. Place it open-side up in an oven-proof dish. Stuff leftover mixed, chopped vegetables into pepper halves. Place slices of tomato over the top. Cook at 350° F (180° C) for 40 to 50 minutes or until the pepper is soft. Serve with broccoli or another very green vegetable.

Variation: For a change from baked potato, serve with "Potato Puffs" (p. 233).

Stuffed Squash

Preparation time: 30 minutes*
* Does not include presoaking
Serves 4-6

3-4 acorn squash
1/2 cup onion, diced
1/2 cup celery, diced
1/2 cup carrot, diced
1-1/4 cup cooked brown rice
1/2 cup lentils sprouted
1/4 cup raisins (or chopped prunes), presoaked and drained
3 tsp. fresh parsley, minced
1/2 tsp. rubbed sage
1/2 tsp. thyme
1 large clove garlic, crushed

Slice squash lengthwise and remove seeds. Presoak raisins (or chopped prunes) (soak overnight in cold water, or pour boiling water over them and leave for a couple of hours until plump) and add. Combine remaining ingredients and fill squash halves. Cover and bake at 300-325° F (149-163° C) for 1-1/2 hours or until squash is tender. Delicious with carrot sauce in "Cauliflower and Carrot Sauce" (p. 212).

Variation: For a delicious mild flavor, try using 6-8 whole garlic cloves. Crushing the fresh garlic releases its strong aromatic oils, whereas using it uncut imparts a mild taste.

Sweet Potato and Apple Bake

Preparation time: 15 minutes
Cooking time: 1 hour
Serves 2

8 oz. sweet potatoes
2 eating apples, sliced
a little water
a little sugar
allspice (optional)

Cook the sweet potatoes gently in their skins until just cooked. Allow to cool. Slice and put into a baking dish alternating with layers of apple. Over each layer, sprinkle some water and a little sugar (and allspice, if using). Bake at 300-350° F (149-177° C) covered for 20 minutes, then remove cover and bake for an additional 10 minutes. Serve as a main dish with a salad (if omitting the allspice) or as a dessert (if using allspice).

Tangy Sweet and Sour Casserole

Preparation time: 20 minutes
Cooking Time: 1-1/2 to 2 hours
Serves 2

1 large (or 2 small) cooking apples
a few slices of leek
1 small onion
1 small sweet potato
1 small parsnip
bay leaf
1 tomato
1 large clove garlic
thyme
1 small zucchini, sliced

Peel and slice the apple, and arrange half the slices in the bottom of a casserole dish. Slice the leek and arrange on top of the apple. Peel and slice the onion and add a layer. Slice the sweet potato, core and chop the parsnip and add a further layer, intermingling with the rest of the apple slices. Put a bay leaf in the middle of the casserole. Skin the tomato and slice, adding a further layer to the casserole. Crush the garlic and sprinkle over the tomato with the thyme and add a layer of sliced zucchini. Cover and bake in the oven at 350° F (180° C) for 1-1/2 to 2 hours.

Vegetable Casserole

Preparation time: 20 minutes
Cooking time: 1 hour

onions
tomatoes
leeks
potatoes
zucchinis
peppers
carrots

Using a heavy saucepan with a tight-fitting lid, slice a layer of either onions, tomatoes or leeks (or all three) and put layer in the bottom of the pan. Take an assortment of sliced, chopped or cubed vegetables and put in layers until about 3/4 full. Add a little water if needed. Cook gently for 45 minutes or until done.

Winter Vegetable Casserole

Preparation time: 20 minutes
Cooking time: 2 hours
Serves 2

sweet potato
parsnip
swede (rutabaga)
celery root
celery stalks
fennel root

tomatoes
Brussels sprouts
bay leaves
water (or soup stock)
fresh parsley, chopped

Chop, slice or dice any or all of the above ingredients (with the exception of the Brussels sprouts and parsley). Put into a large casserole dish with the bay leaves and very little water (or soup stock) to stop the vegetables from sticking. Cover and cook slowly at 325° F (170° C) for 1-1/2 hours. Trim and halve the Brussels sprouts, add to the casserole and continue to cook for another 1/2 hour. Sprinkle with fresh, chopped parsley just before serving.

Zucchini and Potato Bake

Preparation time: 20 minutes
Cooking time: 1-1/2 hours
Serves 2

1 lb. zucchini
1 lb. potatoes
2 medium onions
2 cloves garlic
10 oz. yogurt
fresh parsley, chopped

Finely slice the zucchini, potatoes and onions. Place alternate layers of zucchini, potatoes and onions in a casserole dish, adding a sprinkling of crushed garlic between the layers. Cook in the oven at 300-350° F (149-177° C) for about 1-1/2 hours. Meanwhile, crush the second garlic clove and add to the yogurt. When the dish is cooked, remove from the oven and spread the yogurt mixture on top. Sprinkle chopped fresh parsley over the top and serve immediately.

Zucchini with Garlic and Parsley

Preparation time: 15 minutes
Cooking time: 35 minutes
Serves 2

1 lb. zucchini
3 tbsp. parsley
2 cloves garlic
juice of 1 lemon
flaxseed oil

Chop both ends off the zucchinis and cook whole. While they are cooking, finely chop the parsley and crush the garlic. Mix with the lemon juice and flaxseed oil. Put into a serving bowl. When the zucchinis are cooked, halve lengthwise (if small) or slice thickly (if large). While still hot, add to the serving bowl and toss in the mixture. Serve immediately with oven-roasted bell peppers, a baked potato and a green salad.

Zucchini with Mint

Preparation time: 10 minutes
Cooking time: 30 minutes
Serves 2

4 small zucchinis
2 tbsp. apple cider vinegar
2 tbsp. water
2 tbsp. chopped mint

Cook the zucchinis gently until just cooked but firm. Cut both ends off, then cut diagonally into thin slices. Put into a small casserole dish. Mix the apple cider vinegar, water and chopped mint and pour over the sliced zucchini. Bake gently in the oven at 300° F (149° C) until warmed through. Cool and serve with a baked potato and a green salad.

Desserts

Applesauce, Cooked

Preparation time: 10 minutes
Cooking time: 15-20 minutes
Serves 2

3 medium apples, pared, cored and sliced
honey (or sugar), if needed

Put apple slices in saucepan half covered with cold water. Add honey (or sugar) to taste. Boil about 15 minutes or until soft. Put through food mill.

Applesauce, Fresh

Preparation time: 10 minutes

3 medium apples, pared, cored and sliced
honey (or sugar)

Add honey (or sugar) to taste. Run apples through the grinder portion of the juicer.

Apple Spice Cake

1/4 cup honey (or maple syrup)
1 cup fresh applesauce
1-1/2 cups oat flour
3/4 cup triticale flour
3/4 cup sugar
a pinch of allspice
a pinch of mace
1/4 tsp. coriander
2 cups raisins (or chopped dates)

Crumb topping:
2/3 cup rolled oats
1/3 cup maple syrup (or honey)

a pinch of allspice
a pinch of mace

Combine honey (or maple syrup), applesauce and flours. Sift together sugar, allspice, mace and coriander. Add raisins (or dates). Combine wet and dry ingredients. Pour into nonstick oblong bake pan. For crumb topping, buzz oats briefly in blender to make a finer flake. Mix spices with oats. Mix in enough maple syrup (or honey) to make a crumbly mixture. When the crumb topping is made, sprinkle on top. Bake at 325° F (163° C) for 40 minutes or until cake tests done. Serve with a spoonful of fresh applesauce or yogurt.

Apple-Sweet Potato Pudding

Preparation time: 20 minutes
Cooking time: 30 minutes
Serves 2-3

1 sweet potato, boiled, peeled and sliced
1 apple, raw, peeled and sliced
1 tsp. raisins
1/2 cup bread crumbs
1 tsp. sugar
1/2 cup orange juice
3 tsp. yogurt

Place sweet potato slices in baking dish with apple slices and raisins spread with bread crumbs, sugar and orange juice. Bake in oven at 350° F (177° C) for 30 minutes. Serve hot with yogurt.

Banana (Broiled)

Preparation time: 5 minutes
Cooking time: 10 minutes
Serves 1

1 banana
1 tsp. sugar
lemon juice

Cut banana in half lengthwise and add sugar and a few drops of lemon. Place in pan and broil under low flame in its skin for 10 minutes. Serve hot.

Cherries (Stewed)

Preparation time: 10 minutes
Cooking time: 12 minutes
Serves 2

1/2 lb. cherries, stemmed
1 tsp. potato starch
2 tsp. cold water
2 tsp. sugar (if needed)

Place cherries in saucepan with water to cover. Cook 10 minutes over low flame. Add potato starch dissolved in cold water. Add to boiling cherries. Cook 2 minutes longer. Chill and serve. (Cherries are particularly healthful and are best enjoyed raw.)

Currants

Preparation time: 5 minutes
Serves 1-2

1/4 lb. red currants
3 tsp. sugar
yogurt

Clean currants thoroughly before removing stems. Place in dish, add sugar and serve. Yogurt, sweetened with sugar, may be used for sauce.

Fruit Combination

Preparation time: 5 minutes
Cooking time: 13-15 minutes
Serves 3

3 cups fresh cherries and apricots, halved, sliced and pitted
2 cups water

1/2 cup sugar

2 tsp. cornstarch, dissolved in 1/3 cup cold water

Place fruit with water and sugar in saucepan. Boil gently and slowly for 10 minutes. Add cornstarch. Cook 3 minutes longer. Cool and serve.

Glazed Pear Halves

Preparation time: 15 minutes
Cooking time: 15 minutes
Serves 4

4-5 ripe pears

4 oz. water

4 tbsp. honey (or sucanat, an organic dried cane sugar)

Cut ripe pears into halves and core. Add water to honey (or sucanat) and mix well. Place pear halves in baking dish and pour sugar mixture over them. Bake in slow oven at 250° F (121° C) until done. Baste with juice if necessary.

Oatmeal Cake

Preparation time: 20 minutes
Cooking time: 45 minutes
Serves 6

4 cups oatmeal (dry oats)

2 carrots, grated or blended

honey and raisins (as desired)

Combine all the above ingredients in a baking dish. Put in the oven without a lid and bake for 45 minutes at 250° F (121° C). Serve with yogurt.

Peaches

Preparation time: 15 minutes
Cooking time: 10 minutes
Serves 1-2

1/2 lb. peaches, skinned
2 tsp. sugar

Place peaches in boiling water for 1/2 minute, drain and peel. Cut in halves. Remove pits and place in saucepan with boiling water to half cover fruit level. Cover. Simmer for 10 minutes. Cool. Add sugar and serve chilled.

Pears

Preparation time: 5 minutes
Cooking time: 20 minutes
Serves 1

1 large pear, peeled, cored and halved
1 tsp. sugar

Place pear halves in saucepan with water to half cover. Add sugar and cook for 20 minutes

Plums

Preparation time: 10 minutes
Cooking time: 15 minutes
Serves 1

1/2 lb. plums
2 tsp. sugar

Cut plums in half and remove pits (or plums can be cooked whole). Place in saucepan with water to cover. Cook 15 minutes. Remove, cool and add sugar. Serve chilled.

Prune and Banana Whip

*Preparation time: 10 minutes**
Does not include presoaking
Cooking time: 10 minutes
Serves 2

1 cup dried prunes
2 small bananas, mashed
juice of 1/4 lemon
1 tsp. sugar

Presoak the prunes (soak overnight in cold water, or pour boiling water over them and leave for a couple of hours until plump) and cook for 10 minutes. Whip all ingredients together thoroughly and put in refrigerator for 1 hour. May be served in slices decorated with sweetened yogurt.

Prunes and Apricots (Dried)

*Preparation time: 5 minutes**
* *Does not include presoaking*
Cooking time: 15 minutes
Serves 2

1/2 lb. prunes
1/2 lb. apricots
1/3 cup barley

Presoak the prunes and apricots (soak overnight in cold water, or pour boiling water over them and leave for a couple of hours until plump). Use same water and let boil for 10 minutes or until barley is done. Cool and serve.

Gerson Materials Resource List

A number of items used routinely in the course of the Gerson treatment are not readily available in drug stores, pharmacies, food stores, etc. In order to help persons using this treatment, we suggest the following list. Sources frequently need to be updated. An updated list will be found on the Internet (www.Gerson.org).

Recommended Juicers

Chapter 9, "Juice Machines," in *Healing the Gerson Way*. Also please note that citrus juices (orange or grapefruit) must be extracted with a reamer type, electric or hand operated machine, in order to avoid pressing the skins of oranges, lemons, or grapefruit.

The best juicer for the Gerson Therapy is the Norwalk Hydraulic Press Juicer. All juicers can be configured for export with 220-240 volts.

Contact: Richard Boger, Norwalk Factory Representative
U.S. phone: (800) 405-8423
Overseas phone: +1 (760) 436-9684
www.nwjcal.com

Gerson Therapy Information, Books, DVDs, Videotapes, etc.

Gerson Health Media
316 Mid Valley Center
Carmel, CA 93923
Phone: (831) 625-3565
Fax: (831) 625-9331
E-mail: info@gersonmedia.com
Website: www.gersonmedia.com

The Gerson Institute
P.O. Box 161358
San Diego, CA 92176
Phone: (619) 685-5353
Toll Free in U.S. (888) 4-GERSON (4437766)
Fax: (619) 685-5363
E-mail: info@gerson.org
Website: www.gerson.org

Healing the Gerson Way is now available in:

- Arabic
- Croatian
- German
- Hungarian
- Italian
- Japanese
- Korean
- Polish
- Romanian
- Slovenian
- Spanish

Dr. Max Gerson: Healing the Hopeless is now available in German. Please check for availability with the Gerson Health Media or the Gerson Institute.

For Italian information please contact Margaret Straus
E-mail: margaret.straus@fastwebnet.it

Gerson Health Centre, Hungary
2099 Dobogókö
Téry Ödön u. 18
Hungary
Phone: 0036 30 64 26 341
E-mail: info@gerson.hu
Website: www.gerson.hu

Hungarian Gerson Support Group
Egeszsegforras Alapitvany 1092
Budapest Raday u.37, III.1, Hungary
Phone: 00 36 1 217 1360
E-mail: info@efa.t-online.hu

Singapore

Therapeuolife Education Day Centre (EDC) provides a six-day Gerson Therapy education program, where cancer patients can experience the full Gerson Therapy during the day, Monday through Saturday.

Phone: +65 9002 7443/ +65 9777 8394
Fax: +65 7266163
E-mail: jervinlim@therapeuolife.com
Website: www.therapeuolife.com

Gerson Treatment Medical Supplies

Online

Stat-MX.com
416 W. San Ysidro Blvd.
Suite L-229
San Diego, CA 92173
Phone: (626) 737-0324
Fax: (619) 428-4474
E-mail: stat@stat-mx.com

S.T.A.T., S.A.
Apartado Postal No. 404
Admon. de Correos
Playas de Tijuana, B.C.N. 22501
Mexico
Phone: +(52) 664 680-1103 (Mexico)
Fax: +(52) 664 680-2529 (Mexico)

or

SERVICIOS
Apartado Postal No. 404
Admon. de Correos
Playas de Tijuana, B.C.N. 22501 Mexico
Phone: +(52) 664 680-1103 (Mexico)
Fax: +(52) 664 680-2529 (Mexico)

Checks, Bank drafts, International Bank draft, MasterCard, Visa and Discover cards accepted.

STAT-MX.com supplies Gerson medications; use SERVICIOS as supplier of prescription items, such as needles, crude liver (when available), and B_{12}.

ISHI: Director: Ana Ma. Orozco
524 W. Calle Primera Rd., Suite 1005-E
San Ysidro, CA 92173
866-LAB-ISHI or (866) 522-4744
Phone: (619) 428-6085
Fax: (619) 428-6095

The Key Company
1313 West Essex Avenue
St. Louis, MO 63122
Phone for U.S. & Canada only: (800) 325-9592
General phone: (314) 965-6699
Website: www.thekeycompany.com

For those that want to implement Gerson Therapy
or follow a Gerson lifestyle, who are not located near
a grocery store or farm co-op that offers organic
produce or supplies, there is an option that may be
right for you: The Green Polka Dot Box™. Please
visit www.greenpolkadotbox.com/gersonmedia.

The Green Polka Dot Box is poised to become the largest and most
influential organic buying community ever created. By combining the
delivery of healthy and natural organic foods to health-minded
consumers at affordable prices, with the ability to ship to every zip
code, The Green Polka Dot Box has put an end to the "organic
deserts" that exist throughout America.

Organic Coffee

Royal Blue Organics/Café MAM
P.O. Box 21123
Eugene, OR 97402
Phone: (888) Café-Mam or (888) 223-3626
(541) 338-9585
Website: www.cafemam.com

Information about Fresh Organic Produce

Center for Science in the Public Interest
(provides a list of U.S. mail-order businesses that sell organic food)
1875 Connecticut Avenue NW, Suite 300
Washington, DC 20009-5728
Phone: (202) 332-9110
Website: www.cspinet.org

Co-Op America
(publishes National Green Pages listing businesses
offering organic food)
2100 M Street NW, Suite 403
Washington, DC 20037
Phone: (202) 872-5307
Website: www.coopamerica.org

Diamond Organics
(ships organic produce via FedEx)
1272 Highway 1
Moss Landing, CA 95039
Phone: (888) ORGANIC or (888) 674-2642 or (831) 763-9677
Website: www.diamondorganics.com

Organic Dried Fruit

International Harvest, Inc.
Bob Sterling, Owner
71-40 242nd Street
Douglaston, NY 11362
Phone: (800) 277-4268
Warehouse: (914) 631-3165

Flaxseed Oil

Omega Nutrition
(state that you are a Gerson patient to receive a discount)
6515 Aldrich Road
Bellingham, WA 98226
Ordering: (800) 661-FLAX or (800) 661-3529
Website: www.omeganutrition.com

Water Distillers

The Cutting Edge
Jules Klapper, Owner
P.O. Box 4158
Santa Fe, NM 87502
Phone: (800) 497-9516 or (505) 982-2688
Website: http://cutcat.com

H2Only Distillers
J.C. Smith, Owner
216 Patterson Avenue
Butler, PA 16001
(724) 287-5555 or (800) 4H2Only
Website: www.road-to-health.com/supplements/
h2only_water_distillers.htm

Renewed Health Supply
5106 Ainsworth Drive
Greensboro, NC 27410
Phone: (800) 678-9151 or (336) 460-7678
Website: www.renewedhealth.com

Aqua Clean MD-4
3725 Touzalin Avenue
Lincoln, NE 68507
(contact main office for local Aqua Clean distributor)

Shower Filters

The Cutting Edge
Jules Klapper, Owner
P.O. Box 4158
Santa Fe, NM 87502
Phone: (800) 497-9516 or (505) 982-2688
Website: http://cutcat.com

Sprite Industries, Inc.
1791 Railroad Street
Corona, CA 92880
Phone: (800) 327-9137 or (951) 735-1015
Fax: (951) 735-1016
Website: www.spritewater.com

Ozone Generators and Air Purifiers

The Cutting Edge
Jules Klapper, Owner
P.O. Box 4158
Santa Fe, NM 87502
Phone: (800) 497-9516 or (505) 982-2688
Website: http://cutcat.com

Stainless Steel Enema Buckets

Health & Yoga
(shipped from India)
E-mail: Prakasini@healthandyoga.com
Approximate cost: $30 plus shipping
Website: www.healthandyoga.com/html/product/
enemaequipment.html

Reference Material

Books and Booklets

Healing the Gerson Way, Charlotte Gerson with Beata Bishop (Carmel, CA: Totality Books, 2010). Based on the research of Dr. Max Gerson, this well-written, easy-to-understand, how-to guide for using the Gerson Therapy shows you how to overcome cancer and chronic disease.

Healing Arthritis the Gerson Way, Charlotte Gerson (Carmel, CA: Gerson Health Media, 2012). A complete how-to guide for repairing and reversing arthritic conditions using the well-known Gerson Therapy. Written in an easy-to-read style, it includes the latest medical research on arthritis and updated information on the most common forms of the disease.

Healing Diabetes: The Gerson Way, Charlotte Gerson (Carmel, CA: Gerson Health Media, 2012). This book provides a powerful program to reverse type 2 diabetes and return you to complete health. It offers an easy-to-follow, how-to guide for using the Gerson Therapy to overcome type 2 diabetes, and the simple, step-by-step instructions guide you through each part of the program.

Lose Weight the Gerson Way, Charlotte Gerson (Carmel, CA: Gerson Health Media, 2012). Learn how to lose weight easily, naturally and permanently by using the proven and internationally known Gerson Therapy—an all-natural, nutrition-building and detoxification program that will empower you to lose weight and keep it off for good!

Healing High Blood Pressure the Gerson Way, Charlotte Gerson (Carmel, CA: Gerson Health Media, 2012). Based on the work of Dr. Max Gerson, this book describes the Gerson Therapy—the most powerful and effective system for permanently reducing high blood pressure, opening clogged arteries, lowering elevated blood pressure, losing weight, reducing stress and returning to complete health.

A Cancer Therapy: Results of Fifty Cases and The Cure of Advanced Cancer by Diet Therapy: A Summary of Thirty Years of Clinical Experimentation, Max Gerson, MD (San Diego: Gerson Institute, 2002). Dr. Gerson's seminal work on his cancer therapy, developed over 35 years of clinical experience.

Dr. Max Gerson: Healing the Hopeless, Howard Straus (Carmel, CA: Totality Books, 2009). The official biography of Dr. Max Gerson, chronicling his life and the intertwined development of his therapy, flight from the Nazi Holocaust and struggle against American allopathic medicine.

Censured for Curing Cancer: The American Experience of Dr. Max Gerson, S. J. Haught (San Diego: Gerson Institute, 1991). An investigative reporter who set out to expose Dr. Gerson as a cancer quack, but discovered who the quacks really were.

The Cancer Industry: Unraveling the Politics, Ralph W. Moss (New York: Paragon House, 1989). An exposé of the money and power politics, which drives the industry that it treats and victimizes the cancer patient.

Questioning Chemotherapy, Ralph W. Moss (Brooklyn: Equinox Press, 2000). An analysis of the practice and results of chemotherapy, and the reasons behind its widespread use despite its dismal record.

Death by Modern Medicine, Carolyn Dean, MD (Belleville, Ontario: Matrix Vérité, 2005). Dr. Dean painstakingly gathered government statistics and medical journal data, and published information to show that the #1 killer in the United States is … our medical system.

The China Study: Startling Implications for Diet, Weight Loss and Long-term Health, T. Colin Campbell, PhD, and Thomas M. Campbell II, MD (Dallas: BenBella Books, 2006). One of the world's leading nutritionist sets out his tightly reasoned, experimentally proven case for avoiding animal products, the #1 carcinogen in the world.

Living Proof: A Medical Mutiny, Michael Gearin-Tosh (London: Simon & Schuster UK, Ltd., 2002). An Oxford Don, faced with certain death from multiple myeloma or its allopathic treatments, chooses instead to use the Gerson Therapy and Chinese meditation, and survives his prognosis by over 10 years. Witty, incisive and readable.

Fats That Heal, Fats That Kill, Udo Erasmus (Vancouver, BC: Alive Books, January 1989). The definitive book on fats and oils, and their structures, sources, uses and effects on human health and physiology. Excellent reference.

Fluoride: the Aging Factor, John Yiamouyiannis (Delaware, OH: Health Action Press, 1993). A survey of the suppressed literature on fluoridation of water, vitamins, toothpaste and dental treatments. Chilling and vital information to protect your health and that of your loved ones.

The Root Canal Cover-Up, George Meinig (Ojai, CA: Bion Publishing, 1994). Root canal specialist and cofounder of the American Association of Endontists (root canal specialists) writes about the powerful negative effects of root canals on human health. A must read.

What Really Causes Schizophrenia, Harold D. Foster (Victoria, BC: Trafford Publishing, 2003). Professor Foster presents a novel analysis of the sources and cure of schizophrenia, viewing it as a deficiency or nutritional problem rather than a mental defect.

What Really Causes AIDS, Harold D. Foster (Victoria, BC: Trafford Publishing, 2002). Professor Foster shows the true cause of AIDS as a deficiency of selenium and that it is curable with the proper diet plus selenium supplementation.

Healing booklets by Charlotte Gerson (Carmel, CA: Cancer Research Wellness Institute, 2002; also available from the Gerson Institute, San Diego), 30 pages each. This is a series of nine booklets, eight of which detail the reason why cancer occurs, how and why the Gerson Therapy heals, a short outline of the Gerson Therapy, and about a dozen stories of recovered patients. The ninth booklet covers "Auto-Immune Diseases."

- *Healing Breast Cancer the Gerson Way*
- *Healing Prostate and Testicular Cancer the Gerson Way*
- *Healing Ovarian and Female Organ Cancer the Gerson Way*
- *Healing Colon, Liver and Pancreas Cancer the Gerson Way*
- *Healing Lung Cancer & Respiratory Diseases the Gerson Way*
- *Healing Lymphoma the Gerson Way*
- *Healing Melanoma the Gerson Way*
- *Healing Brain and Kidney Cancer the Gerson Way*
- *Healing "Auto-immune" Diseases the Gerson Way*

Doctor Max (Italian), Giuliano Dego (Barrytown, NY: Station Hill Press, 1997; available from Gerson Institute, San Diego, California). This biographical novel is a broad fictional saga based on the life and times of medical giant Dr. Max Gerson, developer of the Gerson Therapy. One of Italy's leading poets, and winner of the Italian National Paperback Book Prize for this book, Dr. Dego spent decades researching this opus.

Gerson Movies on DVD and Blu-ray

The Beautiful Truth DVD, Stephen Kroschel (Haines, AK: Kroschel Films, 2008). Follow Garrett on a cross-country road trip to investigate the Gerson Therapy where he meets with cancer survivors who present their stories of triumph and healing by following the Gerson Therapy. Garrett also interviews scientists, doctors and researchers who reveal that it is in the best interest of the multibillion dollar medical industry to dismiss the notion of alternative and natural cures.

Dying to Have Known DVD, Stephen Kroschel (Haines, AK: Kroschel Films, 2006). Awarded Honorable Mention, Feature-length documentary category, 2006 New York International Independent Film and Video Festival, New York City, NY. Kroschel presents the testimonies of patients, scientists, surgeons and nutritionists who testify to the Gerson Therapy's efficacy in reversing cancer and other degenerative diseases and present hard, scientific proof to back up their claims.

The Gerson Miracle DVD, Stephen Kroschel (Haines, AK: Kroschel Films, 2004). Winner of the 2004 Golden Palm for "Best Picture," Beverly Hills Film Festival, Beverly Hills, CA. This film introduces Dr. Max Gerson, who developed a proven remedy for cancer and most chronic and degenerative diseases more than 80 years ago. The Gerson Therapy employs a diet and detoxification regimen to rebuild the immune system and restore the body's own ability to heal itself.

The Gerson Movie Collection on Blu-ray. All three Gerson movies on one Blu-ray disc: *The Beautiful Truth, Dying to Have Known* and *The Gerson Miracle.*

Author Index

Subject Index

abdominal edema, 123

abscisic acid, 124

acid reflux, medications not given during, 125

acidol pepsin, 125, 134

Actos, side effects of, 6

acupuncture, 137

adrenaline, produced by aggression, 131

adult-onset diabetes. *See* age-onset (type 2) diabetes

aerosols, 87, 98

affirmations, 162

age-onset (type 2) diabetes, 4–6, 55, 57–59

aggression, during healing reactions, 131

agricultural chemicals
    as contributor to breaking down body's natural defenses, 28–30
    sprayed nearby, lessening effects of, 91
    toxicity of, 94

agrochemicals. *See* agricultural chemicals

air fresheners, 90

air purifiers, 260
    See also ozone generators

air, toxicity of, 26

Ajinomoto, 34

alcoholic beverages
    consumption of in India, 5
    as contributor to breaking down body's natural defenses, 44–46

as forbidden, 94

when allowed, after therapy, 157

allergic reactions
    to carpeting, 90
    to proteins in soy, 96

allopathic medicine. *See* medications, allopathic

allspice, 109

altered foods, 39–40

alternative medicine, 135–137

aluminum foil, 84

aluminum, in pots and utensils, 83

Alzheimer's disease
    aluminum and, 84
    causes of, 34
    effects of aspartame on, 33

AminoSweet, 34

anemia, vitamin B_{12} and, 124

animal products
    in fast food, 17–18
    fiber content in, 10

animal protein
    as contributor to breaking down body's natural defenses, 42–43
    withholding of, 76

anise, 109

antibiotics
    as cause of diabetes, 55–56
    during Gerson Therapy, 152
    in foods, 94

antioxidants
    curcumin, 7

Item	Qty.	Price	Extended
BOOKS			
Healing the Gerson Way	____	$29.95	____
Healing Arthritis the Gerson Way	____	$19.95	____
Healing Diabetes: The Gerson Way	____	$19.95	____
Lose Weight the Gerson Way	____	$19.95	____
Healing High Blood Pressure the Gerson Way	____	$19.95	____
Dr. Max Gerson: Healing the Hopeless, Second Edition	____	$27.95	____
DVDs and BLU-RAY			
The Beautiful Truth DVD	____	$19.95	____
Dying to Have Known DVD	____	$19.95	____
The Gerson Miracle DVD	____	$19.95	____
The Gerson Movie Collection on Blu-ray	____	$24.95	____
BOOKLETS			
Healing Breast Cancer the Gerson Way	____	$4.95	____
Healing Prostate and Testicular Cancer the Gerson Way	____	$4.95	____
Healing Ovarian and Female Organ Cancer the Gerson Way	____	$4.95	____
Healing Colon, Liver and Pancreas Cancer the Gerson Way	____	$4.95	____
Healing Lung Cancer & Respiratory Diseases the Gerson Way	____	$4.95	____
Healing Lymphoma the Gerson Way	____	$4.95	____
Healing Melanoma the Gerson Way	____	$4.95	____
Healing Brain and Kidney Cancer the Gerson Way	____	$4.95	____
Healing "Auto-immune" Diseases the Gerson Way	____	$4.95	____
Subtotal			____
* Shipping/handling			____
9% sales tax (California residents only)			____
Total			____

* *U.S. only shipping charge of $4 per book, $2 per DVD and $1 per booklet. This is an estimated shipping/ handling charge. Actual charge will be calculated by Gerson Health Media. Federal Express charges extra for next-day deliveries for orders placed on Friday.*

Personal checks and major credit cards accepted.

Name _____

Address _____

City/State/Zip _____

Credit Card Number _____ Exp. Date_____

Gerson Health Media
316 Mid Valley Center #230, Carmel, CA 93923
(831) 625-3565 • info@gersonmedia.com • www.gersonmedia.com

Now also available from Gerson Health Media (use order form on overleaf)

 Healing the Gerson Way, Charlotte Gerson with Beata Bishop. Based on the research of Dr. Max Gerson, this well-written, easy-to-understand, how-to guide for using the Gerson Therapy shows you how to overcome cancer and chronic disease. Also included are hints and tips, and more than 90 pages of Gerson-approved recipes.

$29.95

 Healing Arthritis the Gerson Way, Charlotte Gerson. A complete how-to guide for repairing and reversing arthritic conditions using the well-known Gerson Therapy. Written in an easy-to-read style, it includes the latest medical research on arthritis and updated information on the most common forms of the disease.

$19.95

 Healing Diabetes: The Gerson Way, Charlotte Gerson. This book provides a powerful program to reverse type 2 diabetes and return you to complete health. It offers an easy-to-follow, how-to guide for using the Gerson Therapy to overcome type 2 diabetes, and the simple, step-by-step instructions guide you through the program.

$19.95

 Lose Weight the Gerson Way, Charlotte Gerson. Learn how to lose weight easily, naturally and permanently by using the proven and internationally known Gerson Therapy—an all-natural, nutrition-building and detoxification program that will empower you to lose weight and keep it off for good!

$19.95

 Healing High Blood Pressure the Gerson Way, Charlotte Gerson. Based on the work of Dr. Max Gerson, this book describes the Gerson Therapy—the most powerful and effective system for permanently reducing high blood pressure, lowering elevated blood pressure, losing weight, reducing stress and returning to complete health.

$19.95

 Dr. Max Gerson: Healing the Hopeless, by Howard Straus with Barbara Marinacci. Inspiring and uplifting biography of the originator of the Gerson Therapy, chronicling Dr. Gerson's life, development of his world-famous dietary therapy, flight from the Nazi Holocaust and successful search for a holistic and effective treatment for cancer.

$27.95

 The Beautiful Truth DVD, Stephen Kroschel. Follow Garrett on a cross-country road trip to investigate the Gerson Therapy. He meets with cancer survivors who present their stories of triumph and healing by following the Gerson Therapy, and interviews scientists, doctors and researchers who discuss the multibillion dollar medical industry.

$19.95

 Dying to Have Known DVD, Stephen Kroschel. Hear the testimonies of patients, scientists, surgeons and nutritionists who testify to the Gerson Therapy's efficacy in reversing cancer and other degenerative diseases and present hard, scientific proof to back up their claims. Testimonies include a Japanese medical school professor who cured himself of liver cancer over 20 years ago.

$19.95

 The Gerson Miracle DVD, Stephen Kroschel. This film introduces Dr. Max Gerson, who developed a proven remedy for cancer and most chronic and degenerative diseases more than 80 years ago. The Gerson Therapy employs a diet and detoxification regimen to rebuild the immune system and restore the body's own ability to heal itself.

$19.95

 The Gerson Movie Collection on Blu-ray. All three Gerson movies on one Blu-ray disc:
• The Beautiful Truth
• Dying to Have Known
• The Gerson Miracle

$24.95

 Gerson Health Media
316 Mid Valley Center #230, Carmel, CA 93923
(831) 625-3565 • info@gersonmedia.com • www.gersonmedia.com

Item	Qty.	Price	Extended
BOOKS			
Healing the Gerson Way	_____	$29.95	_____
Healing Arthritis the Gerson Way	_____	$19.95	_____
Healing Diabetes: The Gerson Way	_____	$19.95	_____
Lose Weight the Gerson Way	_____	$19.95	_____
Healing High Blood Pressure the Gerson Way	_____	$19.95	_____
Dr. Max Gerson: Healing the Hopeless, Second Edition	_____	$27.95	_____
DVDs and BLU-RAY			
The Beautiful Truth DVD	_____	$19.95	_____
Dying to Have Known DVD	_____	$19.95	_____
The Gerson Miracle DVD	_____	$19.95	_____
The Gerson Movie Collection on Blu-ray	_____	$24.95	_____
BOOKLETS			
Healing Breast Cancer the Gerson Way	_____	$4.95	_____
Healing Prostate and Testicular Cancer the Gerson Way	_____	$4.95	_____
Healing Ovarian and Female Organ Cancer the Gerson Way	_____	$4.95	_____
Healing Colon, Liver and Pancreas Cancer the Gerson Way	_____	$4.95	_____
Healing Lung Cancer & Respiratory Diseases the Gerson Way	_____	$4.95	_____
Healing Lymphoma the Gerson Way	_____	$4.95	_____
Healing Melanoma the Gerson Way	_____	$4.95	_____
Healing Brain and Kidney Cancer the Gerson Way	_____	$4.95	_____
Healing "Auto-immune" Diseases the Gerson Way	_____	$4.95	_____
Subtotal			_____
* Shipping/handling			_____
9% sales tax (California residents only)			_____
Total			_____

* *U.S. only shipping charge of $4 per book, $2 per DVD and $1 per booklet. This is an estimated shipping/ handling charge. Actual charge will be calculated by Gerson Health Media. Federal Express charges extra for next-day deliveries for orders placed on Friday.*

Personal checks and major credit cards accepted.

Name _____

Address _____

City/State/Zip _____

Credit Card Number _____ Exp. Date_____

Gerson Health Media
316 Mid Valley Center #230, Carmel, CA 93923
(831) 625-3565 • info@gersonmedia.com • www.gersonmedia.com

Healing the Gerson Way, Charlotte Gerson with Beata Bishop. Based on the research of Dr. Max Gerson, this well-written, easy-to-understand, how-to guide for using the Gerson Therapy shows you how to overcome cancer and chronic disease. Also included are hints and tips, and more than 90 pages of Gerson-approved recipes.

$29.95

Healing Arthritis the Gerson Way, Charlotte Gerson. A complete how-to guide for repairing and reversing arthritic conditions using the well-known Gerson Therapy. Written in an easy-to-read style, it includes the latest medical research on arthritis and updated information on the most common forms of the disease.

$19.95

Healing Diabetes: The Gerson Way, Charlotte Gerson. This book provides a powerful program to reverse type 2 diabetes and return you to complete health. It offers an easy-to-follow, how-to guide for using the Gerson Therapy to overcome type 2 diabetes, and the simple, step-by-step instructions guide you through the program.

$19.95

Lose Weight the Gerson Way, Charlotte Gerson. Learn how to lose weight easily, naturally and permanently by using the proven and internationally known Gerson Therapy—an all-natural, nutrition-building and detoxification program that will empower you to lose weight and keep it off for good!

$19.95

Healing High Blood Pressure the Gerson Way, Charlotte Gerson. Based on the work of Dr. Max Gerson, this book describes the Gerson Therapy—the most powerful and effective system for permanently reducing high blood pressure, lowering elevated blood pressure, losing weight, reducing stress and returning to complete health.

$19.95

Dr. Max Gerson: Healing the Hopeless, by Howard Straus with Barbara Marinacci. Inspiring and uplifting biography of the originator of the Gerson Therapy, chronicling Dr. Gerson's life, development of his world-famous dietary therapy, flight from the Nazi Holocaust and successful search for a holistic and effective treatment for cancer.

$27.95

The Beautiful Truth DVD, Stephen Kroschel. Follow Garrett on a cross-country road trip to investigate the Gerson Therapy. He meets with cancer survivors who present their stories of triumph and healing by following the Gerson Therapy, and interviews scientists, doctors and researchers who discuss the multibillion dollar medical industry.

$19.95

Dying to Have Known DVD, Stephen Kroschel. Hear the testimonies of patients, scientists, surgeons and nutritionists who testify to the Gerson Therapy's efficacy in reversing cancer and other degenerative diseases and present hard, scientific proof to back up their claims. Testimonies include a Japanese medical school professor who cured himself of liver cancer over 20 years ago.

$19.95

The Gerson Miracle DVD, Stephen Kroschel. This film introduces Dr. Max Gerson, who developed a proven remedy for cancer and most chronic and degenerative diseases more than 80 years ago. The Gerson Therapy employs a diet and detoxification regimen to rebuild the immune system and restore the body's own ability to heal itself.

$19.95

The Gerson Movie Collection on Blu-ray. All three Gerson movies on one Blu-ray disc:
• The Beautiful Truth
• Dying to Have Known
• The Gerson Miracle

$24.95

Gerson Health Media
316 Mid Valley Center #230, Carmel, CA 93923
(831) 625-3565 • info@gersonmedia.com • www.gersonmedia.com